Marcia Hill
Ellyn Kaschak
Editors

For Love or Money:
The Fee in Feminist Therapy

For Love or Money: The Fee in Feminist Therapy has been co-published simultaneously as *Women & Therapy,* Volume 22, Number 3 1999.

*Pre-publication
REVIEWS,
COMMENTARIES,
EVALUATIONS . . .*

"**M**oney seems to be the last taboo in our society. Many people seem to find it easier to talk about their sexual exploits than about how much money they have or earn. This book opens the door and sheds some light and some fresh air onto the topic of money in the therapy relationship. It will engage you and challenge your mind."

Kayla Miriyam Weiner, PhD
*Independent Practice
Seattle, WA*

"**T**he complex meanings of money and specifically the professional fee in the psychotherapeutic relationship are examined from many perspectives in this exciting and timely book about, what the editor calls, 'the last taboo'.

These chapters provide wide-ranging, stimulating analyses of gender, race, class, socioeconomic, clinical setting and other influences on the exchange of money for therapy. Thoughtful case examples add excellent clarity to many of these issues. The emergence of the influential managed care programs, with their critical impact on how payments are made for the delivery of mental health services, have had far-reaching consequences on the meaning of fees. This book is another leading-edge contribution of feminist therapists to psychotherapy literature and is recommended reading for both new and seasoned professionals."

Carolyn C. Larsen, PhD
Senior Counsellor Emeritus
University of Calgary
Partner, Alberta Psychological
Resources Ltd.,
Calgary, Alberta, Canada
Co-editor, Ethical Decision Making in Therapy: Feminist Perspectives

"**H**ill and Kaschak have made a meaningful contribution toward a topic usually known only to female therapists, their accountants, and the IRS: the income of those therapists. The volume helps readers understand why discussing money generally is so difficult for women. Specifically, discussing fees and changes in fees with clients and the resulting issues such a discussion arouses are also explored by the writers. Especially helpful were the vignettes around fee issues; each of them provide the reader an opportunity to evaluate similar experiences."

Elizabeth J. Rave, EdD
Professor of School Psychology
and Women's Studies Emeritus
University of Northern Colorado
Greeley, Colorado

"It is difficult to review such a thought-provoking book in a paragraph. This book aptly points out the complicated area of fee setting and implementation. It questions us valuing ourselves as women and professionals. Issues around fees reflect gender values and conditioning in terms of time, priorities and self-regard.

I like how Marcia Hill and Ellyn Kaschak draw the links between the caring for human suffering that our profession evokes, and the economic realities and decisions and subsequent contradictions of our times."

Annette U. Selmer, MS, LPC
*Portland Counseling
and Psychotherapy Associates
Portland, Oregon*

"The core topic of this edited volume is money: its myriad meanings, its pleasures and pitfalls, and the complex roles, both concrete and symbolic, that money plays in the therapeutic relationship. As helping professionals, most of us have had little training in dealing with the intricate ways in which money can affect the progress and quality of our practice. The chapters in this useful volume cover some of the complex issues involved in how to determine our professional fees and the rationale for reducing the fee; payment for missed appointments; barter in return for service; issues for minority group clients; and the conflicting meanings that money holds for all of us. The contributions range across empirical studies, case examples, a useful review of managed care policies as they impact services for women, and a touching account of how fees infused the relationship between a doctoral student and her imprisoned young client."

Judith Worell, PhD
*Professor Emeritus
University of Kentucky
Lexington, KY*

For Love or Money:
The Fee in Feminist Therapy

For Love or Money: The Fee in Feminist Therapy has been co-published simultaneously as *Women & Therapy,* Volume 22, Number 3 1999.

The *Women & Therapy* Monographic "Separates"

Below is a list of "separates," which in serials librarianship means a special issue simultaneously published as a special journal issue or double-issue *and* as a "separate" hardbound monograph. (This is a format which we also call a "DocuSerial.")

"Separates" are published because specialized libraries or professionals may wish to purchase a specific thematic issue by itself in a format which can be separately cataloged and shelved, as opposed to purchasing the journal on an on-going basis. Faculty members may also more easily consider a "separate" for classroom adoption.

"Separates" are carefully classified separately with the major book jobbers so that the journal tie-in can be noted on new book order slips to avoid duplicate purchasing.

You may wish to visit Haworth's website at . . .

http://www.haworthpressinc.com

. . . to search our online catalog for complete tables of contents of these separates and related publications.

You may also call 1-800-HAWORTH (outside US/Canada: 607-722-5857), or Fax: 1-800-895-0582 (outside US/Canada: 607-771-0012), or e-mail at:

getinfo@haworthpressinc.com

For Love or Money: The Fee in Feminist Therapy, edited by Marcia Hill, EdD, and Ellyn Kaschak, PhD (Vol. 22, No. 3, 1999). *"Recommended reading for both new and seasoned professionals . . . . An exciting and timely book about 'the last taboo' . . . ." (Carolyn C. Larsen, PhD, Senior Counsellor Emeritus, University of Calgary; Partner, Alberta Psychological Resources Ltd., Calgary, and Co-editor, Ethical Decision Making in Therapy: Feminist Perspectives)*

Beyond the Rule Book: Moral Issues and Dilemmas in the Practice of Psychotherapy, edited by Ellyn Kaschak, PhD, and Marcia Hill, EdD (Vol. 22, No. 2, 1999). *"The authors in this important and timely book tackle the difficult task of working through . . . conflicts, sharing their moral struggles and real life solutions in working with diverse populations and in a variety of clinical settings . . . . Will provide psychotherapists with a thought-provoking source for the stimulating and essential discussion of our own and our profession's moral bases." (Carolyn C. Larsen, PhD, Senior Counsellor Emeritus, University of Calgary; Partner, Alberta Psychological Resources Ltd., Calgary, and Co-editor, Ethical Decision Making in Therapy: Feminist Perspectives)*

Assault on the Soul: Women in the Former Yugoslavia, edited by Sara Sharratt, PhD, and Ellyn Kaschak, PhD (Vol. 22, No. 1, 1999). *Explores the applications and intersections of feminist therapy, activism, and jurisprudence with women and children in the former Yugoslavia*

Learning from Our Mistakes: Difficulties and Failures in Feminist Therapy, edited by Marcia Hill, EdD, and Esther D. Rothblum, PhD (Vol. 21, No. 3, 1998). *"A courageous and fundamental step in evolving a well-grounded body of theory and of investigating the assumptions that unexamined, lead us to error." (Teresa Bernardez, MD, Training and Supervising Analyst, The Michigan Psychoanalytic Council)*

Feminist Therapy as a Political Act, edited by Marcia Hill, EdD (Vol. 21, No. 2, 1998). *"A real contribution to the field. . . . A valuable tool for feminist therapists and those who want to learn about feminist therapy." (Florence L. Denmark, PhD, Robert S. Pace Distinguished Professor of Psychology and Chair, Psychology Department, Pace University, New York, New York)*

Breaking the Rules: Women in Prison and Feminist Therapy, edited by Judy Harden, PhD, and Marcia Hill, EdD (Vol. 20, No. 4 & Vol. 21, No. 1, 1998). *"Fills a long-recognized gap in the psychology of women curricula, demonstrating that feminist theory can be made relevant to the practice of feminism, even in prison." (Suzanne J. Kessler, PhD, Professor of Psychology and Women's Studies, State University of New York at Purchase)*

Children's Rights, Therapists' Responsibilities: Feminist Commentaries, edited by Gail Anderson, MA, and Marcia Hill, EdD (Vol. 20, No. 2, 1997). *"Addresses specific practice dimensions that will help therapists organize and resolve conflicts about working with children, adolescents, and their families in therapy." (Feminist Bookstore News)*

More than a Mirror: How Clients Influence Therapists' Lives, edited by Marcia Hill, EdD (Vol. 20, No. 1, 1997). *"Courageous, insightful, and deeply moving. These pages reveal the scrupulous self-examination and self-reflection of conscientious therapists at their best. AN IMPORTANT CONTRIBUTION TO FEMINIST THERAPY LITERATURE AND A BOOK WORTH READING BY THERAPISTS AND CLIENTS ALIKE." (Rachel Josefowitz Siegal, MSW, retired feminist therapy practitioner; Co-Editor, Women Changing Therapy; Jewish Women in Therapy; and Celebrating the Lives of Jewish Women: Patterns in a Feminist Sampler)*

Sexualities, edited by Marny Hall, PhD, LCSW (Vol. 19, No. 4, 1997). *"Explores the diverse and multifaceted nature of female sexuality, covering topics including sadomasochism in the therapy room, sexual exploitation in cults, and genderbending in cyberspace." (Feminist Bookstore News)*

Couples Therapy: Feminist Perspectives, edited by Marcia Hill, EdD, and Esther D. Rothblum, PhD (Vol. 19, No. 3, 1996). *Addresses some of the inadequacies, omissions, and assumptions in traditional couples' therapy to help you face the issues of race, ethnicity, and sexual orientation in helping couples today.*

A Feminist Clinician's Guide to the Memory Debate, edited by Susan Contratto, PhD, and M. Janice Gutfreund, PhD (Vol. 19, No. 1, 1996). *"Unites diverse scholars, clinicians, and activists in an insightful and useful examination of the issues related to recovered memories." (Feminist Bookstore News)*

Classism and Feminist Therapy: Counting Costs, edited by Marcia Hill, EdD, and Esther D. Rothblum, PhD (Vol. 18, No. 3/4, 1996). *"EDUCATES, CHALLENGES, AND QUESTIONS THE INFLUENCE OF CLASSISM ON THE CLINICAL PRACTICE OF PSYCHOTHERAPY WITH WOMEN." (Kathleen P. Gates, MA, Certified Professional Counselor, Center for Psychological Health, Superior, Wisconsin)*

Lesbian Therapists and Their Therapy: From Both Sides of the Couch, edited by Nancy D. Davis, MD, Ellen Cole, PhD, and Esther D. Rothblum, PhD (Vol. 18, No. 2, 1996). *"Highlights the power and boundary issues of psychotherapy from perspectives that many readers may have neither considered nor experienced in their own professional lives." (Psychiatric Services)*

Feminist Foremothers in Women's Studies, Psychology, and Mental Health, edited by Phyllis Chesler, PhD, Esther D. Rothblum, PhD, and Ellen Cole, PhD (Vol. 17, No. 1/2/3/4, 1995). *"A must for feminist scholars and teachers . . . These women's personal experiences are poignant and powerful." (Women's Studies International Forum)*

Women's Spirituality, Women's Lives, edited by Judith Ochshorn, PhD, and Ellen Cole, PhD (Vol. 16, No. 2/3, 1995). *"A delightful and complex book on spirituality and sacredness in women's lives." (Joan Clingan, MA, Spiritual Psychology, Graduate Advisor, Prescott College Master of Arts Program)*

Psychopharmacology from a Feminist Perspective, edited by Jean A. Hamilton, MD, Margaret Jensvold, MD, Esther D. Rothblum, PhD, and Ellen Cole, PhD (VOl. 16, No. 1, 1995). *"Challenges readers to increase their sensitivity and awareness of the role of sex and gender in response to and acceptance of pharmacologic therapy." (American Journal of Pharmaceutical Education)*

Wilderness Therapy for Women: The Power of Adventure, edited by Ellen Cole, PhD, Esther D. Rothblum, PhD, and Eve Erdman, MEd, MLS (Vol. 15, No. 3/4, 1994). *"There's an undeniable excitement in these pages about the thrilling satisfaction of meeting challenges in the physical world, the world outside our cities that is unfamiliar, uneasy territory for many women. If you're interested at all in the subject, this book is well worth your time." (Psychology of Women Quarterly)*

Bringing Ethics Alive: Feminist Ethics in Psychotherapy Practice, edited by Nanette K. Gartrell, MD (Vol. 15, No. 1, 1994). *"Examines the theoretical and practical issues of ethics in feminist therapies. From the responsibilities of training programs to include social issues ranging from racism to sexism to practice ethics, this outlines real questions and concerns." (Midwest Book Review)*

Women with Disabilities: Found Voices, edited by Mary Willmuth, PhD, and Lillian Holcomb, PhD (Vol. 14, No. 3/4, 1994). *"These powerful chapters often jolt the anti-disability consciousness and force readers to contend with the ways in which disability has been constructed, disguised, and rendered disgusting by much of society."* (Academic Library Book Review)

Faces of Women and Aging, edited by Nancy D. Davis, MD, Ellen Cole, PhD, and Esther D. Rothblum, PhD (Vol. 14, No. 1/2, 1993). *"This uplifting, helpful book is of great value not only for aging women, but also for women of all ages who are interested in taking active control of their own lives."* (New Mature Woman)

Refugee Women and Their Mental Health: Shattered Societies, Shattered Lives, edited by Ellen Cole, PhD, Oliva M. Espin, PhD, and Esther D. Rothblum, PhD (Vol. 13, No. 1/2/3, 1992). *"The ideas presented are rich and the perspectives varied, and the book is an important contribution to understanding refugee women in a global context."* (Comtemporary Psychology)

Women, Girls and Psychotherapy: Reframing Resistance, edited by Carol Gilligan, PhD, Annie Rogers, PhD, and Deborah Tolman, EdD (Vol. 11, No. 3/4, 1991). *"Of use to educators, psychotherapists, and parents–in short, to any person who is directly involved with girls at adolescence."* (Harvard Educational Review)

Professional Training for Feminist Therapists: Personal Memoirs, edited by Esther D. Rothblum, PhD, and Ellen Cole, PhD (Vol. 11, No. 1, 1991). *"Exciting, interesting, and filled with the angst and the energies that directed these women to develop an entirely different approach to counseling."* (Science Books & Films)

Jewish Women in Therapy: Seen But Not Heard, edited by Rachel Josefowitz Siegel, MSW, and Ellen Cole, PhD (Vol. 10, No. 4, 1991). *"A varied collection of prose and poetry, first-person stories, and accessible theoretical pieces that can help Jews and non-Jews, women and men, therapists and patients, and general readers to grapple with questions of Jewish women's identities and diversity."* (Canadian Psychology)

Women's Mental Health in Africa, edited by Esther D. Rothblum, PhD, and Ellen Cole, PhD (Vol. 10, No. 3, 1990). *"A valuable contribution and will be of particular interest to scholars in women's studies, mental health, and cross-cultural psychology."* (Contemporary Psychology)

Motherhood: A Feminist Perspective, edited by Jane Price Knowles, MD, and Ellen Cole, PhD (Vol. 10, No. 1/2, 1990). *"Provides some enlightening perspectives. . . . It is worth the time of both male and female readers."* (Comtemporary Psychology)

Diversity and Complexity in Feminist Therapy, edited by Laura Brown, PhD, ABPP, and Maria P. P. Root, PhD (Vol. 9, No. 1/2, 1990). *"A most convincing discussion and illustration of the importance of adopting a multicultural perspective for theory building in feminist therapy. . . . THIS BOOK IS A MUST FOR THERAPISTS and should be included on psychology of women syllabi."* (Association for Women in Psychology Newsletter)

Fat Opression and Psychotherapy, edited by Laura S. Brown, PhD, and Esther D. Rothblum, PhD (Vol. 8, No. 3, 1990). *"Challenges many traditional beliefs about being fat . . . A refreshing new perspective for approaching and thinking about issues related to weight."* (Association for Women in Psychology Newsletter)

Lesbianism: Affirming Nontraditional Roles, edited by Esther D. Rothblum, PhD, and Ellen Cole, PhD (Vol. 8, No. 1/2, 1989). *"Touches on many of the most significant issues brought before therapists today."* (Newsletter of the Association of Gay & Lesbian Psychiatrists)

Women and Sex Therapy: Closing the Circle of Sexual Knowledge, edited by Ellen Cole, PhD, and Esther D. Rothblum, PhD (Vol. 7, No. 2/3, 1989). *"ADDS IMMEASUREABLY TO THE FEMINIST THERAPY LITERATURE THAT DISPELS MALE PARADIGMS OF PATHOLOGY WITH REGARD TO WOMEN."* (Journal of Sex Education & Therapy)

The Politics of Race and Gender in Therapy, edited by Lenora Fulani, PhD (Vol. 6, No. 4, 1988). *Women of color examine newer therapies that encourage them to develop their historical identity.*

Treating Women's Fear of Failure, edited by Esther D. Rothblum, PhD, and Ellen Cole, PhD (Vol. 6, No. 3, 1988). *"SHOULD BE RECOMMENDED READING FOR ALL MENTAL HEALTH PROFESSIONALS, SOCIAL WORKERS, EDUCATORS, AND VOCATIONAL COUNSELORS WHO WORK WITH WOMEN."* (The Journal of Clinical Psychiatry)

Women, Power, and Therapy: Issues for Women, edited by Marjorie Braude, MD (Vol. 6, No. 1/2, 1987). *"RAISE[S] THERAPISTS' CONSCIOUSNESS ABOUT THE IMPORTANCE OF CONSIDERING GENDER-BASED POWER IN THERAPY. . . welcome contribution.'' (Australian Journal of Psychology)*

Dynamics of Feminist Therapy, edited by Doris Howard (Vol. 5, No. 2/3, 1987). *"A comprehensive treatment of an important and vexing subject.'' (Australian Journal of Sex, Marriage and Family)*

A Woman's Recovery from the Trauma of War: Twelve Responses from Feminist Therapists and Activists, edited by Esther D. Rothblum, PhD, and Ellen Cole, PhD (Vol. 5, No. 1, 1986). *"A MILESTONE. In it, twelve women pay very close attention to a woman who has been deeply wounded by war.'' (The World)*

Women and Mental Health: New Directions for Change, edited by Carol T. Mowbray, PhD, Susan Lanir, MA, and Marilyn Hulce, MSW, ACSW (Vol. 3, No. 3/4, 1985). *"The overview of sex differences in disorders is clear and sensitive, as is the review of sexual exploitation of clients by therapists. . . . MANDATORY READING FOR ALL THERAPISTS WHO WORK WITH WOMEN.'' (British Journal of Medical Psychology and The British Psychological Society)*

Women Changing Therapy: New Assessments, Values, and Strategies in Feminist Therapy, edited by Joan Hamerman Robbins and Rachel Josefowitz Siegel, MSW (Vol. 2, No. 2/3, 1983). *"An excellent collection to use in teaching therapists that reflection and resolution in treatment do not simply lead tp adaptation, but to an active inner process of judging.'' (News for Women in Psychiatry)*

Current Feminist Issues in Psychotherapy, edited by The New England Association for Women in Psychology (Vol. 1, No. 3, 1983). *Addresses depression, displaced homemakers, sibling incest, and body image from a feminist perspective.*

For Love or Money:
The Fee
in Feminist Therapy

Marcia Hill, EdD
Ellyn Kaschak, PhD
Editors

For Love or Money: The Fee in Feminist Therapy has been co-published simultaneously as *Women & Therapy,* Volume 22, Number 3 1999.

The Haworth Press, Inc.
New York • London • Oxford

For Love or Money: The Fee in Feminist Therapy has been co-published simultaneously as *Women & Therapy*™, Volume 22, Number 3 1999.

The Haworth Press, Inc., 10 Alice Street, Binghamton, NY 13904-1580 USA

Library of Congress Cataloging-in-Publication Data

For love or money : the fee in feminist therapy : Marcia Hill, Ellyn Kaschak, editors.
    p. cm.
    "For love or money : the fee in feminist therapy has been co-published simultaneously as women & therapy, Volume 22, number 3, 1999."
    Includes bibliographical references and index.
    ISBN 0-7890-0955-2 (alk. paper)–ISBN 0-7890-0956-0 (alk. paper)
    1.Feminist therapy–Miscellanea. 2. Psychotherapists–Fees. 3. Psychotherapist and patient.
I. Hill, Marcia. II. Kaschak, Ellyn, 1943-
RC489.F45 F67 1999
616.89′14′082–dc21
                                                                    99-051402

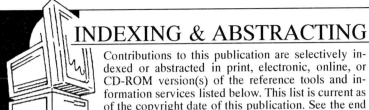

INDEXING & ABSTRACTING

Contributions to this publication are selectively indexed or abstracted in print, electronic, online, or CD-ROM version(s) of the reference tools and information services listed below. This list is current as of the copyright date of this publication. See the end of this section for additional notes.

- *Abstracts of Research in Pastoral Care & Counseling*

- *Academic Abstracts/CD-ROM*

- *Academic Index (on-line)*

- *Alternative Press Index*

- *Behavioral Medicine Abstracts*

- *BUBL Information Service, an Internet-based Information Service for the UK higher education community <URL: http://bubl.ac.uk/>*

- *CNPIEC Reference Guide: Chinese National Directory of Foreign Periodicals*

- *Contemporary Women's Issues*

- *Current Contents: Clinical Medicine/Life Sciences (CC: CM/LS) (weekly Table of Contents Service), and Social Science Citation Index. Articles also searchable through Social SciSearch, ISI's online database and in ISI's Research Alert current awareness service*

- *Digest of Neurology and Psychiatry*

- *Expanded Academic Index*

- *Family Studies Database (online and CD/ROM)*

- *Family Violence & Sexual Assault Bulletin*

- *Feminist Periodicals: A Current Listing of Contents*

- *GenderWatch*

- *Health Source: Indexing & Abstracting of 160 selected health related journals, updated monthly*

(continued)

- *Health Source Plus: expanded version of "Health Source"*

- *Higher Education Abstracts*

- *IBZ International Bibliography of Periodical Literature*

- *Index to Periodical Articles Related to Law*

- *Mental Health Abstracts (online through DIALOG)*

- *ONS Nursing Scan in Oncology-NAACOG's Women's Health Nursing Scan*

- *PASCAL, c/o Institute de L'Information Scientifique et Technique. Cross-disciplinary electronic database covering the fields of science, technology & medicine. Also available on CD-ROM.*

- *Periodical Abstracts, Research I, general & basic reference indexing & abstracting data-base from University Microfilms International (UMI)*

- *Periodical Abstracts, Research II, broad coverage indexing & abstracting data-base from University Microfilms International (UMI)*

- *Psychological Abstracts (PsycINFO)*

- *Published International Literature on Traumatic Stress (The PILOTS Database)*

- *Sage Family Studies Abstracts (SFSA)*

- *Social Work Abstracts*

- *Sociological Abstracts (SA)*

- *Studies on Women Abstracts*

- *Violence and Abuse Abstracts: A Review of Current Literature on Interpersonal Violence (VAA)*

- *Women Studies Abstracts*

- *Women's Studies Index (indexed comprehensively)*

(continued)

Special Bibliographic Notes related to special journal issues (separates) and indexing/abstracting:

- indexing/abstracting services in this list will also cover material in any "separate" that is co-published simultaneously with Haworth's special thematic journal issue or DocuSerial. Indexing/abstracting usually covers material at the article/chapter level.
- monographic co-editions are intended for either non-subscribers or libraries which intend to purchase a second copy for their circulating collections.
- monographic co-editions are reported to all jobbers/wholesalers/approval plans. The source journal is listed as the "series" to assist the prevention of duplicate purchasing in the same manner utilized for books-in-series.
- to facilitate user/access services all indexing/abstracting services are encouraged to utilize the co-indexing entry note indicated at the bottom of the first page of each article/chapter/contribution.
- this is intended to assist a library user of any reference tool (whether print, electronic, online, or CD-ROM) to locate the monographic version if the library has purchased this version but not a subscription to the source journal.
- individual articles/chapters in any Haworth publication are also available through the Haworth Document Delivery Service (HDDS).

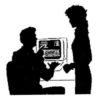

ABOUT THE EDITORS

Marcia Hill, EdD, is a psychologist who has spent over 25 years practicing psychotherapy. She is co-editor of the journal *Women & Therapy* and a member and past Chair of the Feminist Therapy Institute. In addition to therapy, Dr. Hill does occasional teaching, writing, and consulting in the areas of feminist therapy theory and practice. The Editor of *More than a Mirror: How Clients Influence Therapists' Lives* (1997) and *Feminist Therapy as a Political Act* (1998), she has co-edited five other Haworth books: *Classism and Feminist Therapy: Counting Costs* (1996); *Couples Therapy: Feminist Perspectives* (1996); *Children's Rights, Therapists' Responsibilities: Feminist Commentaries* (1997); *Breaking the Rules: Women in Prison and Feminist Therapy* (1998) and *Learning from Our Mistakes: Difficulties and Failures in Feminist Therapy* (1999). She is currently in private practice in Montpelier, Vermont.

Ellyn Kaschak, PhD, is Professor of Psychology at San Jose State University in San Jose, California. She is author of *Engendered Lives: A New Psychology of Women's Experience*, as well as numerous articles and chapters on feminist psychology and psychotherapy. She has had thirty years of experience practicing psychotherapy, is past Chair of the Feminist Therapy Institute and of the APA Committee on Women and is Fellow of Division 35, the Psychology of Women, Division 12, Clinical Psychology, Division 45, Ethnic Minority Issues and Division 52, International Psychology, of the American Psychological Association. She is co-editor of the journal *Women & Therapy.*

For Love or Money:
The Fee in Feminist Therapy

CONTENTS

For Love *and* Money

Marcia Hill

Burdened by childhood anxieties and silenced by the myth of a classless society, the fee in psychotherapy has been a source of too much discomfort and too little discussion. We hover between hunger and generosity, guilt and resentment. Earning a living is well and good, but what kind of living, with how much luxury? Women therapists particularly, socialized to prioritize others' needs, may be painfully mindful that we earn a living from the suffering of others. In the short step from empathizing with our clients to identifying with our clients, we find ourselves considering that we take a vacation or make an extravagant purchase that our clients could not afford, using money that represents the sacrifices they make to pay for therapy. Because the exchange of money in therapy takes place in an intimate context, therapists, especially those paid directly by their clients, are faced daily with questions about economic injustice in a way that those who work for a paycheck are not.

Sex was the taboo topic in Freud's time; talk about money is the forbidden in ours. Do you know your friends' incomes? Those of your family members? The amount of savings, if any, they have? Do you know what your colleagues charge? How much they earn? How many clients they see at a reduced fee? Both having and not having money can be a source of shame, with those having less money feeling inadequate and those with more wanting to hide their privilege. The wish to earn a substantial income in the human service field is often consid-

The author thanks Tim Sargent and Shari Stahl for a lively discussion about fees that informed much of this paper.

[Haworth co-indexing entry note]: "For Love *and* Money." Hill, Marcia. Co-published simultaneously in *Women & Therapy* (The Haworth Press, Inc.) Vol. 22, No. 3, 1999, pp. 1-3; and: *For Love or Money: The Fee in Feminist Therapy* (eds: Marcia Hill, and Ellyn Kaschak) The Haworth Press, Inc., 1999, pp. 1-3. Single or multiple copies of this article are available for a fee from The Haworth Document Delivery Service [1-800-342-9678, 9:00 a.m. - 5:00 p.m. (EST). E-mail address: getinfo@haworthpressinc.com].

ered crass: we should work for love, the money is incidental. We should not work for love *and* money.

If we are in private practice, our autonomy as a business person is constrained by clinical pressures. We are responsible for collecting copayments which are frequently unaffordable; in an effort to meet the market, that obligation is widely ignored. As a result, we as therapists hold the tension between the market realities and our legal obligations. We wish to be available to a wide range of people, so we join "preferred provider" networks; the result is that our clients pay less out of pocket but we are also reimbursed at a lower rate. Our clients rarely know this, and we hold the tension between our wish to make therapy accessible and wanting to earn our full fee. Because the costs of doing business in psychotherapy are generally invisible, our fees may look inflated to the client; and again, we carry the tension between needing to earn something over our expenses and appearing avaricious.

The frustrations of being self-employed apply to other professions as well as to psychotherapists, but for us they carry the added emotional impact of the therapy relationship's closeness and meaning. A client who does not pay her/his bill has stolen from me, yet pursuing legal redress has therapeutic implications, and can leave one open to malpractice lawsuits as well. Yet, if I run across a former client who hasn't paid me several years after therapy ended, my first thought will be "She owes me money," followed by discomfort with my pettiness. Remembering this unpaid bill for all that time is a testament to my frustration, and feeling ashamed of my anger is a testament to the message that I should caretake people for love only.

No discussion of money in psychotherapy can ignore the effects of managed care on therapists' ability to earn a living. In general, the public is unaware that at least some managed care "benefits" are in fact losses to the clinician. I have heard a number of therapists confide that they don't mean to sound paranoid, but wonder whether insurance requirements are designed to make clinicians give up on being paid. Requirements for detailed paperwork and preauthorization are easy to lose track of, and sharply higher error rates (mysteriously and inevitably in the insurer's favor) in reimbursement checks can mean repeated calls to insurance companies in an effort to correct the mistakes. Virtually every clinician has stories of money earned but lost for such reasons. What does this do to our ability to accept pro bono or reduced fee clients? What does it do to our love of our work? I have heard therapists express frustration that their job description must now include fighting to be paid for their work.

We do work for love: for the love of our clients and the miracle of the process of transformation. But we work also for money: to earn a living and, yes, to have some luxury in our lives. The work of a therapist includes what is perhaps the most complex relationship possible between labor and income. We are certainly not paid for what we produce, and there is not even a direct relationship between our time and our earnings. Between the two comes a convoluted array of variables. These include the personal, such as our ability to set a fair fee or to enforce payment for missed sessions. There are ethical factors, for example, our sense of social responsibility, and clinical considerations, such as the meaning of the fee to the client. Organizational limits and requirements–those of the insurers–are figured in as well. It is not surprising that we are confused.

Nonetheless, money is a substantial part of how we get fed by our work. It is part of what protects us from expecting emotional return from our clients. Our income thus is not only what we take from our labor, it is what enables us to give. We work for love *and* money.

Psychotherapists' Ambivalence About Fees: Male-Female Differences

Ella Lasky

SUMMARY. This article focuses on the mixed feelings that psychotherapists have about setting fees. It highlights the different conflicts that male and female therapists have about fees. Sixty psychotherapists were interviewed and these results are presented as well as vignettes illustrating five typical therapist conflicts.

KEYWORDS. Male, female, gender, psychotherapists, money, fees

Many psychotherapists are ambivalent about setting fees. In general, very little attention has been paid to psychologists' feelings about

Ella Lasky, PhD, has written numerous articles about women's self esteem, women's achievement conflicts, and women's feelings about their physical attractiveness. She is in private practice in New York City and is a supervisor of individual and family therapy in several doctoral programs and institutes in the New York metropolitan area.

Address correspondence to: Ella Lasky, 865 West End Avenue, 1A, New York, NY 10025.

This article is adapted from the original Rosewater, L.B. and Walker, L.E.A. (1985), "Psychotherapists' Ambivalence About Fees," in *Handbook of Feminist Therapy: Women's Issues in Psychotherapy*, New York: Springer Publishing Co. It is adapted with the permission of the publisher.

[Haworth co-indexing entry note]: "Psychotherapists' Ambivalence About Fees: Male-Female Differences." Lasky, Ella. Co-published simultaneously in *Women & Therapy* (The Haworth Press, Inc.) Vol. 22, No. 3, 1999, pp. 5-13; and: *For Love or Money: The Fee in Feminist Therapy* (eds: Marcia Hill, and Ellyn Kaschak) The Haworth Press, Inc., 1999, pp. 5-13.

fee setting in our professional workshops and literature (Canter, 1995; Citron-Bagget & Kempler, 1991; Lasky, 1980, 1981, 1985). Since Freud, there have been numerous articles focused on the techniques of setting fees and on patients' reaction to fees (Herron & Welt, 1992), but not on the therapists' feelings.

To explore the conflicts involved in this issue further, I conducted an informal survey (Lasky, 1985) of 60 psychotherapists from various parts of the country whose experience ranged from 2.5 to 20 years. While not a representative sample, it contains lively and useful anecdotal data that provide the basis for a discussion of this subject. There were dramatic differences between the ways that male and female psychotherapists felt about money and fees.

One fact is certain: Ambivalence about setting fees exists, and it is not confined to novices. Two-thirds of those surveyed expressed considerable intrapsychic conflict about setting fees and establishing the other parameters of the therapeutic contract. The most commonly expressed conflicts involved balancing a sense of professional worth with the necessity to earn a living and the desire to help people. Many therapists feel uncomfortable dealing with the business side of therapy, for they entered the field to facilitate other goals. Some therapists reported feeling like oppressors for wanting to take money from people who are upset and need therapy; others expressed concern that they feel excited, powerful, apologetic, or embarrassed when setting a high fee, and guilty, annoyed, or resentful when setting a low one. Some felt greedy if they refused to work with a particular patient because of his or her inability to pay a reasonable fee; others report that they feel "too good" or "too powerful" when the fees they charge allow them to earn a comfortable living.

Unfortunately, the psychology profession provides little or no training concerning money matters. The reasons why the area of financial management is so blatantly neglected in our training are complex. It may be that psychologists stay away from addressing the issue of money because, like other professionals, we feel it is beneath our dignity. It also may be that, since our training takes place in clinics and hospitals where patients pay a secretary or cashier and not the therapist directly, there is simply no motivation to discuss or adjust fees. The beginning therapist usually feels relieved by this arrangement and typically does not discuss the fee again unless the patient brings the topic up. This is unfortunate, because we are losing a fertile training opportunity by our avoidance of this issue.

The matter of money and what it represents is a challenge to everyone. Our society instills in us conflicting values about money. While the American credo tells us that "we are all created equal," we also learn that "some people (the rich) are more equal than others (the poor)" (Lindgren, 1980). Money has other symbolic meanings which vary from person to person (Walker & Garman, 1992). In general, it is fair to say that money is a taboo subject for everyone in America including psychologists. This is illustrated by the fact that most of us do not know how much money our friends make. Therefore, we learn about money and money issues in an unspoken way, and the individual meanings are determined by each person's life circumstances: the religion, culture, and social class of one's family; the attitude of one's parents toward money; and the way money actually was handled in the family.

There are important differences in the ways men and women approach the issue of making money. These differences are demonstrated by the following studies.

Steven Stein developed a test of Daniel Goleman's Emotional Intelligence Quotient (EQ) and found significant differences in the emotional intelligence of men and women. After studying 7,700 people, Stein found that women score higher than men on measures of empathy and social responsibility, and that men are more able to tolerate stress and are more self-confident than women (reported by Murray, 1998). These findings confirm and explain my findings (see below) that women, because of their higher empathy levels and stronger sense of social responsibility than men, were more likely to lower their fees to patients who seem needy. These findings also confirm and explain my findings that men's higher self-confidence helps them ask for their full fees.

Two recent studies found that both female and male participants believed that men would pay themselves significantly more than women would. The men in the study did, in fact, pay themselves more than the women did. The researchers had hypothesized that these results may have been influenced by the subjects' recent incomes, with those people who had earned higher salaries paying themselves more than the people who earned lower salaries. They controlled for this effect and found that it was not the case. In discussing how they decided what to pay themselves, the men reported wanting to maximize their own financial gains. In addition, the amount they were paid was significantly more important to the men than it was to the women (Desmaris & Curtis, 1997). This replicates the results of Callahan-Levy and Meese (1979) eighteen years earlier.

There are gender differences in how women and men spend, save and handle money. Prince (1993) found that while both genders see money as closely linked with esteem and power, men were more likely to feel involved and competent in money handling and were more willing to take risks to amass wealth. Women, on the other hand, had a greater sense of envy and deprivation with respect to money as a means of obtaining things and experiences that they could enjoy.

In 1998, the average woman continued to earn less than the average man. Women earned 76 cents for every dollar men made during the first quarter of 1998; this is an improvement over 20 years ago when the pay gap between men and women was such that women earned 63 cents for every dollar made by men in 1979 ("Pay Gap," *Wall Street Journal*, 1998). This even applies to doctoral level psychologists with equal training. The salaries of male psychologists with two to four years full time experience were found to be higher than the salaries of women psychologists, with men making $43,050 to women's $41,152 (American Psychological Association, 1998, Table 15B.)

My interviews with psychotherapists in private practice (Lasky, 1985) revealed that 75 percent of the women charge lower fees than men of the same level of experience in their geographic area, 15 percent charge the same fees, and 10 percent charge more than their male peers. Why is it that most of the women psychologists with about the same level of experience would be unable or unwilling to charge the going rate in their area? It may be that many women psychotherapists, like the women in the aforementioned studies, undervalue their professional services or that men overvalue theirs. Other women psychotherapists simply felt that providing excellent professional services was more important to them than earning high fees. Finally, it may be that women may compare themselves to women colleagues and men to men.

Many women therapists are feminist therapists who reflect a humanistic orientation regarding fee setting. One of the key principles of feminist therapy is that the therapist-patient relationship strives to be more egalitarian (Gilbert, 1980). The general consensus today is that the therapy relationship can never be truly egalitarian, but that the feminist therapist strives toward appropriate sharing of power (Feminist Therapy Institute, 1987). In light of this, most feminist therapists use a sliding scale and negotiate a fee that will be fair to both patient and therapist. This is especially important because a goal of feminist therapists is to make professional services accessible to as wide a range of patients as possible. Women, minority women in particular, are concentrated in lower-paying jobs and therefore would suffer from the insistence on a non-negotiable fee.

My interviews indicate that it is particularly difficult for most women psychotherapists to be clear inside themselves about their fees. While two-thirds of both men and women interviewed have conflicts about determining fees, the focus of these conflicts differs. Many men revealed that they glossed over the internal conflict and resolved it by focusing on how much income they needed to support their families. Women psychotherapists, on the other hand, tend to be acutely aware of the conflict about setting fees. They feel a three-way conflict: (1) needing to support themselves and their families, (2) feeling torn between working additional hours to earn more money and wanting to spend the time with their friends and family, and (3) focusing more on the patient's financial needs than on their own. These different conflicts are understandable, since men are responding to years of conditioning to earn money while women only recently have begun to think about it as a choice. Some conflicts about fees that are common among male and female therapists emerged from these interviews.

Therapist Jones is an overly-nurturant female therapist. She agrees to see Ms. A at a fee lower than her usual one. As a result of their work together, Ms. A gets a promotion and raise. When Therapist Jones suggests increasing the fee, Ms. A says she is reluctant to do so. Therapist Jones does not counter her reluctance forcefully and subsequently feels resentful, used, and foolish for having lowered her fee for this patient. When she calms down, she realizes that she has just learned something new about Ms. A's psychodynamics and the way Ms. A treats others. In fact, Therapist Jones realizes that she feels just like Ms. A's lover is often described to feel, and therefore sees that the issue presents a good opportunity to explore with Ms. A how she often tries to manipulate others through her helplessness, greed, self-centeredness, and contempt. Addressing the issue proved fruitful for both the patient and the therapist.

For Therapist Smith the most difficult circumstance regarding fees takes place when a patient, who has created a self-defeating circumstance, asks for a reduction of the fee or number of sessions per week. The patient, Mr. B, recently has arranged a nearly impossible work situation for himself that commits him to longer hours and more travel, thereby reducing the time available for therapy. He asks Therapist Smith to lower the number of sessions per week because of his situation. Therapist Smith finds the request difficult to deal with because she feels manipulated, hurt, and angry. She is uncertain if her reaction is appropriate, and she decides to consult a colleague on the matter. As a result it becomes clear that the patient had a role in creating the problem and can rearrange his work hours and return to the original therapy schedule. When this is pointed out to him, the patient feels relieved. Therapist Smith then uses this opportunity to point out that the way he has treated her relates to the often unilateral way he makes and breaks contracts with other people; she is able to use this event to look at other aspects of his character structure.

Therapist White has a firm approach to fees. He began working with a woman, Ms. C, who could not really afford the fee as set and she did not realize that some therapists offer a sliding scale. Had he paid more attention to her body language when he set the fee he would have known this, but he neglected this and focused on the amount of money he needs to earn. The patient came to therapy for two months, paying the full fee in a timely way and when she could no longer afford this fee she simply ended the treatment. Therapist White had no idea of what happened or why.

Therapist Adams reports taking into treatment at a reduced fee a young man in his late thirties, Mr. D, whose economic resources are limited. After several months, Mr. D brings in some insurance forms and mentions that he hadn't realized he'd had these benefits. He doesn't propose adjusting the fee, and Therapist Adams feels exploited and manipulated. She blames herself for failing to ask about insurance in the initial interview and this self-blame makes it difficult to decide how to handle the situation. Many women therapists are particularly vulnerable to charming, needy young patients who "forget" about their own resources. Some therapists identify with them, others want to love and care for them. Unfortunately, this often leads to unconscious collusion between the patient's style and the therapist, and blocks the patient's progress.

Therapist Green works long hours but doesn't have the commensurate income. She feels she can't ask any of her patients for higher fees because she doesn't want to "burden" them, nor does she want to seem "greedy." Ironically, she has never explored money matters fully with her patients and doesn't know who can or cannot afford higher fees. It is her own reaction formation against greed that stands in the way of a fuller exploration of this issue.

Among the benefits of being clear in your own mind about your fee structure is an ability to be comfortable rather than defensive when you discuss money matters with your patients. This is of significant value to the therapeutic relationship. As we know, almost every patient, no matter what the presenting symptom, has ambivalence about money. By being clear about your own fee you will offer the patient, perhaps for the first time, the refreshing experience of having a frank, open, and unambiguous discussion about money. Second, if your patient is angry about something related to money, your own comfort with the topic may allow you to understand the patient's emotional pain and hostility without appearing defensive, doctrinaire, or apologetic. Finally, setting appropriate fees for your patients will help make it more difficult for them to relax into passively dependent help-seeking.

Setting fees that are too low for a particular patient often will elicit gratitude, humiliation, or shame reactions and may inhibit expressions of hurt, anger, love, or resentment toward the therapist. Fees that are too high often will elicit anger, resentment, humiliation, or shame reactions and often result in premature terminations of therapy. They also may inhibit the expression of dependency, closeness, appreciation, hurt, or love toward the therapist. Establishing your fee structure requires careful thought and consideration. Fees that are either too high or too low can be countertherapeutic.

It is clear that therapists undermine the treatment when they become flustered about their position on fees. These are some practical steps one can take to deal with conflicts about money:

1. Take notice of when and with which types of patients these conflicted feelings arise. Try to assess whether you are being overly nurturant, self-blaming or narcissistic when it comes to setting your fee. After having gathered the data about yourself, you can identify your pattern and then work on each situation as it arises.

2. Include in your initial interview questions about income, assets, expenses, loans, insurance benefits, and so forth. This will set the stage for money to be an ordinary topic of discussion in the therapy and will help in setting a proper fee.
3. Review your caseload and income before a consultation with a potential patient. This will help clarify your decisions about whether to take additional patients and about what kind of patients to take, and will help you to make a rational decision about your fee.
4. Review the cost of running your office. Understand that you do have an overhead, like any other business; this may help you focus on setting fees that are appropriate.
5. Consult with a colleague if it seems that you cannot resolve your fee problems. Occasionally, one might go back into therapy or analysis to explore this issue.

Clarity about what you charge for your professional services has many benefits for your patients and yourself. Among the benefits is the freedom to think and speak about a taboo topic so that it does not control you. This freedom will enhance your sense of professional and personal worth.

REFERENCES

American Psychological Association (1998). *1997 salaries in psychology.* Research Office, American Psychological Association. Washington, DC.

Callahan-Levy, C.M., & Meese, L.A. (1979). Sex differences in the allocation of pay. *Journal of Personality and Social Psychology, 37,* 433-446.

Canter, M.E. (1995). Money and psychotherapy: The female experience. *Psychotherapy in Private Practice, 14,* 29-33.

Citron-Bagget, S. & Kempler, B. (1991). Fee setting: Dynamic issues for therapists in independent practice. *Psychotherapy in Private Practice, 5,* 45-60.

Desmaris, S. and Curtis, J. (1997). Gender and perceived pay entitlement: Testing for effects of experience with income. *Journal of Personality and Social Psychology, 72,* 141-150.

Feminist Therapy Institute. (1987). Feminist therapy code of ethics and ethical guidelines for feminist therapists. Denver: Author.

Gilbert, L.A. (1980). Feminist therapy. In A.M. Brodsky & R.T. Hare-Mustin (Eds.), *Women and psychotherapy* (pp. 245-266). New York: Guilford Press.

Herron, W.G. & Welt, S.R. (1992). *Money matters: The fee in psychotherapy and psychoanalysis.* New York: Guilford Press.

Lasky, E. (1980, September). The therapist as socialized female. Conversation hour at the annual convention of the American Psychological Association, Montreal.

Lasky, E. (1981, March). Money and fees. Conversation hour at the Midwinter Convention of the Psychotherapy Division of the American Psychological Association, San Antonio, TX.

Lasky, E. (1985). Psychotherapists' ambivalence about fees. In L.B. Rosewater and L.E.A. Walker (Eds.). (1985). *Handbook of feminist therapy: Women's issues in psychotherapy.* New York: Springer Press.

Lindgren, H.C. (1980). *Great expectations: The psychology of money.* Los Altos, CA: William Kaufman.

Murray, B. (1998). Does 'emotional intelligence' matter in the workplace? *APA Monitor,* July 1998, p. 21.

"Pay gap between men and women begins to narrow again after a pause." (1998, June 10). *Wall Street Journal,* p. B6.

Prince, M. (1993). Women, men and money styles. *Journal of Economic Psychology, 14,* 175-182.

Walker, R. & Garman, E.T. (1992). The meanings of money: Perspectives from human ecology. *American Behavioral Scientist, 35,* 781-789.

What Are We Worth?
Fee Decisions of Psychologists
in Private Practice

Ruth Parvin
Gail Anderson

SUMMARY. This study consisted of eight interviews done with psychologists in private practice, four female and four male, of European American origin. Their responses to questions about decision making regarding fees provide fertile ground for future research. Psychologists' thoughts about fee-setting and adjustment appear to be complex and widely variable. Although the findings are limited due to sample size and homogeneity, the results suggest that: psychologists may be ambivalent about discussing their fees; managed care practices may be undercutting a willingness of therapists to do pro bono, sliding or adjusted fee work; a gender analysis should include family-of-origin socioeconomic status in fee decisions; women may be considerably more flexible in adjusting fee decisions; psychologists are increasingly eager to find self-pay clients instead of third party pay or managed care pay clients due to the constraints and burdens of such payers; and psychologists are often confused about their ethical and legal mandates pertaining to fee-setting and management. *[Article copies available for a fee from The Haworth Document Delivery Service: 1-800-342-9678. E-mail address: getinfo@haworthpressinc.com <Website: http://www.haworthpressinc.com>]*

Ruth Parvin, JD, PhD, has a private practice in Portland, OR. As a feminist therapist and mediator, Ruth consults and does training on a variety of mental health issues. Gail Anderson, MA, a psychotherapist employed with Lutheran Social Service of Minnesota, particularly enjoys feminist play therapy with children.

The authors wish to express their appreciation to Andrew A. Anderson for his careful reading and suggestions.

Address correspondence to: Gail Anderson, Lutheran Social Service, 26 7th Avenue N, St. Cloud, MN 56303.

[Haworth co-indexing entry note]: "What Are We Worth? Fee Decisions of Psychologists in Private Practice." Parvin, Ruth, and Gail Anderson. Co-published simultaneously in *Women & Therapy* (The Haworth Press, Inc.) Vol. 22, No. 3, 1999, pp. 15-25; and: *For Love or Money: The Fee in Feminist Therapy* (eds: Marcia Hill, and Ellyn Kaschak) The Haworth Press, Inc., 1999, pp. 15-25. Single or multiple copies of this article are available for a fee from The Haworth Document Delivery Service [1-800-342-9678, 9:00 a.m. - 5:00 p.m. (EST). E-mail address: getinfo@haworthpressinc.com].

KEYWORDS. Fees, ethics, gender

Do women and men psychologists think and act differently when making fee determinations? What are the factors which propel our decision-making process about fees? These questions originally motivated our interest in this study. While we were not prepared to conduct a major research project, we decided that interviewing a small sample of psychologists would be worthwhile to elicit themes deserving further consideration. Earlier research had suggested that there were some distinct gender differences in fee determination.

In an informal study of 60 psychotherapists, Lasky (1985) found that two-thirds expressed considerable discomfort about fee-setting. She attributed this discomfort to their original motivation for entering the field: the desire to help others. She suggests that therapists may feel guilt or identification with the oppressor for getting paid because someone is having a hard time coping with life. On the other hand, therapists want to make an adequate income to compensate themselves for their work.

In another study, Lasky (1984) found that 75% of the women therapists charged lower fees than their male colleagues with similar education and experience. Lott (1987) reviewed research findings that women pay themselves less than men for the same work, suggesting that money may be a less salient reward for women than men or that women may be less privy to the standard against which male colleagues measure the value of their work.

In her interviews, Lasky (1984) found that many women had conflicting emotions about fees. They wanted to support themselves and their families and work extra hours for additional money. They also wanted to have those same hours available for family and friends and they tended to be concerned about the cost of therapy on their clients' financial situations. Lasky (1984) found that women attempted to balance their decisions among these factors. In contrast, she discovered that men were more likely to handle any fee-setting issues by figuring out how much money they and their families needed and adjusting their fees to insure this income.

Parvin and Anderson (1995) examined the interaction between feminist values and monetary issues in therapy, observing that in the political analysis of power, the distribution of money is one of the major determinants of who gets health care and therapy. As they pointed out, the client who works for minimum wage may not earn enough in an eight-hour workday to pay for one full fee hour of therapy. Brown (1990) commented that feminist therapists get caught in a bind when they apply a political analysis to the conduct of business because the business of therapy is earning a living by dealing with human pain and despair, often accompanied by a lack of client resources.

METHODS

Participants

Search for Participants

Participants for this study initially came from a comprehensive list of doctoral psychologists licensed for the first time in 1980 and 1990 who practice in a major west coast city. A letter was personally written and addressed to each of the 44 psychologists who met this criteria. Of the three who initially replied, one stated that she was too busy and two agreed to be interviewed. Follow-up calls were made two weeks later which elicited four responses, two of whom agreed to participate, one who wanted to consult an attorney first to ensure that there would be no risk in participating, and one who said she never participated in research studies.

A second follow-up call was made. There were two responses, one who said she would have no time for at least four weeks and she was unwilling to schedule after that time period, and one who said she did not respond to research requests as a policy. Finally, we abandoned our attempt to get a pseudo-scientific sampling and contacted personal acquaintances for help. In six weeks, we had completed eight interviews.

Demographics

Participants had an average length of licensure of 16 years, ranging from nine to 28 years. The average length of practice was almost identical for female and for male psychologists. The sample identified with a full spectrum of theoretical perspectives, with men reporting a slight bias toward cognitive/behavioral schools and women a stronger leaning toward psychodynamic/object relations orientations. Only one woman identified herself as a feminist therapist, although two additional women identified themselves as feminists. Of the women, two identified their family of origin as upper middle class, two as middle class. One man identified his family of origin as upper middle class, one as middle class, one as lower middle and one as working lower middle class.

Workload

Participants were asked how many hours they work a week "doing psychology" which was defined to include consultation, teaching, paperwork, etc. Hours ranged from 25 to 50 per week with women averaging 31 hours per week and men 46 hours per week. They were also asked how many hours of therapy they do weekly. Averages of therapy hours by gender were: females: 24, with a range of 22-25, and males: 17, with a range of 4-32. (One man is an administrator in community mental health with a small private practice on the side and another focuses on evaluations rather than therapy.)

Materials and Procedures

The authors prepared eight questions regarding basic demographic information we considered relevant to the inquiry. In addition, female psychologists were asked if they considered themselves feminist therapists. We also devised a nine-question survey entitled "Past and Current Fee-Setting Procedures." These two sets of questions were the basis for our taped, 20-30 minute interviews.

Questions asked about past and current fee-setting practices were:

1. When you started private practice, how did you decide what to charge?
2. Currently, what is your primary basis for setting fees?
3. Rank the following by their importance to you for fee-setting:
   a. Whether the person has insurance?
   b. What other therapists with your experience charge?
   c. Respect or prestige based on your charge?
   d. What the person can afford to pay?

    e. What the prognosis is for the client? (the projected ability for the therapist and client to work well together and the client to make progress within a certain time frame)

    f. Other?

4. Do you have a sliding fee? How did you make that decision? Under what circumstances and what are the criteria you use for adjusting fees? What percentage of clients do you see on a sliding fee?

5. Has the fee you accept from third party payers affected your current fee practice with private pay clients?

6. Do you currently or have you ever bartered your services? If so, under what conditions?

7. How do you handle fee payment and non-payment? Do you ever use a collection agency?

8. Where do you refer uninsured individuals with minimum pay jobs for therapy and what is the lowest fee charged there?

9. What other questions about fee-setting and adjustments would you like to see researched?

Question 3 was first scored by dividing answers by gender. Each first choice was given a value of six, each second choice a value of five, third choice a value of four, etc. Scores by gender for each factor were added to produce ranking.

All references to a standard fee designate a 50-minute therapy session.

RESULTS

Initial and Current Fee-Setting Practices

Gender differences did not influence initial fee-setting decisions. All participants consulted supervisors, colleagues or agencies and set their initial fees at a rate slightly lower than the market standard, reflecting a desire to build a practice. Current fee-setting decisions were more divergent, although seven of the eight respondents identified that what other therapists with their experience charged remains the primary factor in their fee-setting decisions. One therapist described how his accountant who works with other psychologists consistently encourages him to increase his fees to maintain a fee schedule similar to that of his colleagues. He stated that while he does not personally believe therapy is worth the amount that is charged, he will probably follow this recommendation.

The following factors listed in order of importance were the most influential for both genders for fee-setting and adjustment decisions:

1. what other therapists with your experience charge,
2. what a person can afford to pay, and
3. whether the person has insurance.

Two males and no females endorsed "respect or prestige based on your charge" which was fourth in importance for men. One woman and two men stated that "prognosis for the client" affected their likelihood to make fee adjustments for clients. This factor was fifth in importance for men and fourth in importance to women. One male added the factor of managed care reimbursements as significant to his fee-setting decisions.

Sliding Fee Scales and Adjustments

Seven psychologists accept less than their standard fee from third-party payers. One woman's practice is on a cash-only basis.

Females

No female psychologist has a formal sliding fee, but all adjusted their fees in some cases. The most common reason for fee adjustment was that a client who has been in therapy for a while has a financial setback or runs out of insurance coverage. One therapist estimated that 85% of her cases are paid for by managed care contracts. Managed care pays much less than her standard fee of $110. Thus, she considers her managed care cases to be adjustments to her standard fee. This woman values being available to a diversified clientele and "tithes" a certain number of no or low-cost therapy hours to clients whose insurance has run out. Nonetheless, she is less likely to reduce fees since managed care inception because her standard fee has already been discounted by managed care payment reductions.

Another woman, who acknowledged that she has another income in her family, does not mention a sliding fee initially, but adjusts her standard fee of $95 if a case is referred by a colleague and/or the client makes a clear case for needing a lower fee. She is more willing to do this if the case sounds particularly interesting, or if she feels strongly that she and the client will work well together. About 20% of her clients are on a sliding fee from $5 and up. This woman, of "middle class" origin, is strongly motivated by the belief that she has the ability to help people and that economic issues should not overshadow the importance of the work.

The remaining two women adjust their fees, mostly for clients who have exhausted their insurance benefits. One charges $110 and slides down to $75 for 10% of her clients. The other professional charges $120 but will slide down to $50; 25-30% of her clients are on a reduced fee.

Males

Three of the four male interviewees do not have a sliding or adjustable fee. One male does not adjust his standard fee of $95 because he feels adjustments are too complicated administratively. He does, however, negotiate the payment schedule to allow clients to pay over an extended period of time. He set his fee at a level "where it's at least reachable for someone who does not use third party payment."

Another therapist has a very small private practice; he feels he cannot afford to reduce his fee of $100. His full-time work is in a community agency that does have a sliding fee. He feels that his committee work for professional organizations and the community is a type of pro bono work.

The third interviewee charges $95 and only adjusts his fee for graduate psychology students who pay half-price. He says sliding fees open "too many doors for misunderstanding," i.e., clients who compare may not understand differing rates.

The one male therapist with a sliding fee states that he wishes to be available to those who have limited finances. He mentioned that he grew up in a "low middle class" family where money was tight. Although he normally charges $95, about 25% of his clients pay reduced fees, as low as $50 per session. He also does contract work at a lower fee for community agencies. Custody evaluations which are charged at a higher rate per case ($2000-3000) help cover his lower cost therapy.

Two male interviewees maintained that lower fees from contracts or managed care cut into their ability to have sliding fees. One psychologist felt that lowering rates when insurance runs out subtly encourages insurance companies to cut back on what they offer. He claims one prominent HMO offers inadequate in-house mental health care and supplements it with five-session referrals to a private practice, thus abdicating its responsibility to provide the services needed. Another therapist was concerned that by basing fees on what third party payers will pay "we eventually price ourselves out of reach to more and more people and we become more and more dependent on insurance and other third party payers."

A male respondent commented that a major shift in the practice of psychology is that therapists have taken the responsibility for collecting from the insurance companies. When he started working, the clients were responsible for paying a fee and for procuring their own reimbursement if insurance was involved. One woman mentioned that she is a member of a National Mental Health Alliance which has a toll-free number and a web page offering a 20% discount to clients who accept responsibility for collecting their own third party pay reimbursement or do not use their insurance.

Comparison of Fees and Adjusted Fees by Gender

The women psychologists' average standard fee is $109 and they average 18% of their clients on adjusted fees. By contrast, the average rate for the male psychologists is $98, and only one male adjusts his fee. He adjusts down to as low as $50 for 25% of his clientele. One woman adjusts her fee as low as $5, another adjusts down to $50, another to $75. The fourth woman states she tithes 10% of her hours "at no or low fee."

Bartering

Two women and one man have bartered their services in rare instances where the value of the product (artwork in all cases) was determined prior to the arrangement and no negotiation was necessary. No one saw bartering as a frequent option and five of the interviewees had never bartered, nor did they anticipate doing so. Only one psychologist stated awareness that the American Psychological Association's Ethical Principles of Psychologists and Code of Conduct (1992) has changed toward a very limited permission to use bartering under strictly defined circumstances. One woman had exchanged short-term therapy services for the right to tape the sessions for use in training supervisees.

Fee Payment and Non-Payment

Respondents of both genders seldom use collection agencies. Three men never used collection agencies and the fourth rarely used them. Of the female respondents, one woman had used a collection agency only one time, two rarely used this method (one clarified that she would only use collections after therapy was terminated), and the fourth did not answer the question. Collection agencies were most commonly used after repeated billing and when psychologists felt that clients had been given excellent services and appeared to have the money to pay. Most had a procedure of sending increasingly strongly written letters asking for payment. However, female and male therapists usually wrote off uncollected bills rather than sending them for collection.

Referrals

Therapists were asked how they respond to someone who calls them for therapy who has no insurance and a minimal-wage job. Some do not get these calls due to their answering services. Others indicated they refer to low-cost community agencies or clinics staffed by therapists in training at a local professional psychology or nursing school. Only three of the interviewees (two women and one man) had accurate information about the fees charged at these places. Most significantly underestimated the minimum fees.

DISCUSSION

We found the process of this study as interesting as the content of the interviews. We were surprised at the difficulty we had finding people willing to be interviewed considering the process was anonymous, brief, and in their own offices. While this might have been due to their tight schedules, the interviews took place during the late summer, often a fairly slow time in private practice. We asked our interviewees how they would explain this reluctance.

The general consensus was that therapists are uncomfortable discussing money. Reasons for this might be: psychologists feel competitive with each other and believe that their fee-setting practices are trade secrets, their self-identity as helping professionals seems incongruent with a focus on fees, they are concerned that they might be criticized in print, or that public discussion of fee practices might lead to being scrutinized by insurance companies or condemned by ethics boards.

Some therapists avoid pro bono, sliding or adjusted fee work because they are concerned that it could cause them legal problems. Others offer lower fees for uninsured and low-income clients because they feel it is the right thing to do. However, they worry that if their practices were audited, they could be legally challenged for this practice. Psychologists of both genders expressed a desire to move toward a cash-only or private pay practice and one female had already developed such a practice.

Our study indicates that psychologists want and need guidance in legal and ethical mandates for setting and adjusting fees, matters of collection and other monetary issues in the business of doing therapy. There seemed to be a high level of confusion or disagreement about whether the following are legal and ethical: sliding fees, writing off co-payments which are unpaid because of financial hardship, lowering fees when a client's insurance runs out, and having a different fee schedule for private pay versus third party pay clients. Therapists who had discussed these issues with insurance companies reported getting a wide variety of answers which left them no more assured than before.

We asked our interviewees if they had questions they suggest be researched. One man was most interested in how to set up a cash-only practice. Two women wondered if there is a difference in fee-setting and collection between therapists who are the sole support for themselves or their families and those who have a second income. Another suggested that political party affiliation might predict the answers to some of our questions. One woman wondered if women worked fewer hours than male psychologists (which we found to be true in this study).

CONCLUSIONS

Our purpose was to study fee decisions by gender and to determine some of the factors which are relevant to psychologists in making fee decisions. We found a gender difference in fee adjustment with female psychologists being more flexible and offering a greater percentage of adjustment in their fee policies. However, males in this study offered a lower standard fee than the female interviewees. This finding may be confounded by more of the men in our sample coming from lower to middle class families of origin and more of the women identifying with upper middle to upper income family origin. Women psychologists in this sample worked fewer total hours, and were more likely to focus on therapy instead of work activities such as consultation, assessment and evaluation or administration.

The interrelationship among gender, family-of-origin socioeconomic status, and fee decisions deserves more sophisticated study with a larger, more diverse sample. Other questions we hope to explore in the future include whether fee adjustment correlates with a therapist's enjoyment of working with a particular client and how therapists from different disciplines such a social workers, psychiatric nurses, or professionals identifying as feminist therapists might answer similar questions differently.

REFERENCES

American Psychological Association (1992). *Ethical principles of psychologists and code of conduct.* Washington, DC.

Brown, L.S. (1990). Ethical issues and the business of therapy. In H. Lerman & N. Porter (Eds.), *Feminist ethics in psychotherapy* (pp. 60-69). New York: Springer.

Lasky, E. (1984). Psychoanalysts and psychotherapists: Conflicts about setting fees. *Psychoanalytic Psychology, 4,* 289-300.

Lasky, E. (1985). Psychotherapists' ambivalence about fees. In L.B. Rosewater & L.E.A. Walker (Eds.), *Handbook of feminist therapy: Women's issues in psychotherapy* (pp. 250-256). New York: Springer.

Lott, B. (1987). *Women's lives: Themes and variations in gender learning.* New York: Brooks/Cole.

Parvin, R., & Anderson, G. (1995). Monetary issues. In E.J. Rave & C.C. Larsen (Eds.), *Ethical decision making in therapy: Feminist perspectives* (pp. 57-87). New York: Guilford Press.

Women, Mental Health, and Managed Care: A Disparate System

Claudia G. Pitts

SUMMARY. Managed care has changed the way that mental health care is provided. These insurers manage such factors as length and type of therapy made available, access to therapy, and level of payment for therapy. Women, as the majority of those insured by managed care and as consumers of mental healthcare, are differentially affected by these changes. *[Article copies available for a fee from The Haworth Document Delivery Service: 1-800-342-9678. E-mail address: getinfo@haworthpressinc.com <Website: http://www.haworthpressinc.com>]*

KEYWORDS. Managed care, mental health, psychotherapy, women

With over 70 million enrollees, managed care plans have changed the way that Americans receive health care (National Research Corporation, 1996). Health care consumers have all become quite familiar with the primary care physician as "gatekeeper," limits on the treatment received, and health professionals being managed by the managed care companies. All of these "innovations" were developed to lower health care costs and still provide care to enrollees. Women's

Claudia Pitts, PhD, is a psychologist in private practice in Lake Zurich, Illinois.

Address correspondence to: Claudia Pitts, PhD, 228 West Main Street, Lake Zurich, IL 60047.

[Haworth co-indexing entry note]: "Women, Mental Health, and Managed Care: A Disparate System." Pitts, Claudia G. Co-published simultaneously in *Women & Therapy* (The Haworth Press, Inc.) Vol. 22, No. 3, 1999, pp. 27-36; and: *For Love or Money: The Fee in Feminist Therapy* (eds: Marcia Hill, and Ellyn Kaschak) The Haworth Press, Inc., 1999, pp. 27-36. Single or multiple copies of this article are available for a fee from The Haworth Document Delivery Service [1-800-342-9678, 9:00 a.m. - 5:00 p.m. (EST). E-mail address: getinfo@haworthpressinc.com].

healthcare has become a particular source of controversy within the health care industry. Issues such as hospital stays for mastectomies, pregnancy, and childbirth care, and allowing women to choose their primary care physicians have all become political issues (Kaiser Family Foundation, 1998). Another area of political controversy has been mental healthcare parity (Kaiser Family Foundation, 1998). Women, as the majority of mental healthcare consumers (National Center for Health Statistics, 1997), have been strongly and differentially affected by this lack of parity and other changes wrought by the onset of managed care. In other words, as a service that is used by more women, mental health care is more often restricted and limited than those services equally used by either gender.

MONEY, MENTAL HEALTH AND MANAGED CARE

Insurance coverage, especially under managed care, has traditionally either neglected mental health needs or covered them at significantly lower levels than medical and other health needs. Nowhere are these trends more apparent than in behavioral health care, a division which combines mental health and drug and alcohol treatment, created by the managed care companies (Gonen, 1997).

Typically, a fee-for-service insurance provider pays for health care at an 80% rate with 20% of the charge as a copayment by the insured. Mental health care by fee-for-service providers is typically paid at a 50% rate, with 50% paid by the consumer (Health Care Financing Administration, 1998). Medicare also typically pays only 50% and has additionally instituted the "psychiatric reduction." The approved amount paid for mental health service is already less than the typical clinician's fee. The "psychiatric reduction" causes mental health care to be paid for at half of this approved amount (Health Care Financing Administration, 1998) rather than at the 80% rate approved for other medical services. Fee-for-service insurers, including Medicare, occasionally still offer virtually unlimited mental health care sessions. More often, however, they will cover approximately 20 sessions per year to be used at the discretion of the consumer and the provider (Miller, 1996).

Managed behavioral health care differs significantly from these fee-for-service plans. Although some managed care plans state in their literature to the prospective consumer that there are 20 or more psychotherapy sessions available to them, this is often not actually the case. In fact, the case manager allows sessions in blocks. For example, after three or five sessions, it is incumbent on the provider to call the managed care case manager and persuade them to allow another block of sessions. This process, however, holds risk for both the consumer and the provider. For the consumer, there may be questions of confidentiality if explicit detail is given to the case manager in order to be awarded more sessions. Especially when an employer is very small or when it is self-insured, clients may feel as if the information may not be properly safeguarded. Another hazard can exist if the provider persuades too strongly. A record of "extended psychotherapy" on the medical insurance database may present a block to future insurance. For the provider, records are kept by the managed care company as to average number of sessions per provider and those with high averages may not receive future referrals. However, the hazards of undertreatment, legal, ethical, and psychological, can be more serious to both client and provider. Undertreated clients may feel worse than before treatment. Abbreviated treatment may also discourage those unsatisfied with the treatment from seeking future treatment. Providers may find themselves at risk for having not alleviated the problems that they have been treating. This may result in a conflict, possibly with legal implications, arising between the client and provider.

Payment for behavioral health services within managed care also varies widely. Some managed care organizations (MCOs) integrate behavioral health into overall health care services and include behavioral health providers within their networks. Others contract out to stand-alone behavioral health companies, "carving out" behavioral health services from general medical care. As of 1997, 149 million insured Americans with mental health coverage received their behavioral health services through carve-outs (Gonen, 1997). Although carve-out proponents suggest that specialization in behavioral health increases quality, the continuing division between physical and behavioral health only serves to deepen this schism. Indeed, payment using carve-out programs are often "flat fee" and far below the "usual and customary" rate as the carve-out company profits from money not paid to providers. In other words, if the rate the carve-out company pays the clinician is less than what the carve-out receives from the insurance company, they profit. Reductions in clinician payment increase profit. These sort of reduced payment levels and carve-outs are exclusive to the mental health payment system and may serve to inhibit access to adequate mental health care by managed care enrollees (Miller, 1996).

Virtually all HMOs do offer some outpatient mental health benefits. Less than two percent (1.5%) of all HMOs do not offer any outpatient mental health care and just over two percent (2.3%) deny coverage of inpatient mental health care. Copayments, the per session payment by the client, vary considerably. Nearly twenty-seven percent (26.6%) of plans offer the option of zero copayments and 22.3 percent require a $20 copayment (Group Health Association of America, 1995). These payments are considerably lower than the 50% typically required by fee-for-service insurers. However, these savings may dim when the number of sessions authorized is quite low. In some situations, the client then pays at 100% for any sessions beyond the number authorized.

Sliding scale payments made available by private therapists might seem to be a remedy to these problems. However, therapists that accept any insurance benefits are often restricted in their ability to adjust fees for clients. Insurance companies want the lowest price available and can be punitive if a lower fee is being offered to clients and not to them (F. Fields, personal communication, October 10, 1998).

DEMOGRAPHICS

Based on a survey (1995) by the Commonwealth Fund, managed care enrollees are younger, less educated, less affluent, and are more likely to be of African-American or Hispanic heritage, female and to work in smaller firms than fee-for-service members. Most managed care enrollees (53%) were under age 40, compared with 43% of fee-for-service members in this age group. Twenty-eight percent of managed care enrollees had a high school education or less, compared with 21% of fee-for-service members.

Managed care plans had more low-income enrollees (9%) with annual household earnings of $15,000 or less than fee-for-service plans (5%). Eleven percent of managed care enrollees were African American and 17 percent were Hispanic, compared with 8 percent of African American and 12 percent of Hispanic members in fee-for-service plans. Fifty-five percent of managed care enrollees were women, compared with 51 percent of fee-for-service members. Forty-five percent of managed care enrollees worked in firms with fewer than 500 employees, compared with 37 percent of fee-for-service plan members (Davis, 1996). Managed care insurance packages tend to have less employer cost than fee-for-service plans. Employers of lower paid workers may tend to offer more managed care plans. Ethnic minorities and women are over-represented in this group. The disparity in type of employment and rate of pay may account for some of the difference in the population of these two groups.

"Penetration" into markets by managed care varies widely. High levels are especially apparent in the West (Arizona, California) where over 70 percent of insurance enrollees are involved in HMOs (76.6% Tucson, AZ, 74.2% Sacramento, CA, and 73.1% San Diego). Lower levels tend to cluster in the South with levels of less than ten percent (Jackson, MS, 9.9%, Lafayette, LA, 8.4%) (American Association of Health Plans, 1996).

Insurance which tends to be more heavily regulated, cost controlled and which denies the freedom to choose one's own provider seems to be frequently associated with those in the less affluent sectors of society. This type of stratification of medical insurance suggests differences in accessible health care by class, gender, ethnicity, and geography.

MANAGED CARE AND MENTAL HEALTH

Medication, psychotherapy, or a combination of both can be used to treat many mental health problems. For example, the success rate for the use of medication alone in the treatment of depression is between 60 and 80 percent, with success defined as some improvement (Gonen, 1997). Medications alone, however, are not usually sufficient for effective treatment of depression, and for mild depression, the use of cognitive therapy first is recommended over medication (Gonen, 1997). Managed care organizations have raised some concern in this area. While managed care has helped to increase the number of Americans with mental health coverage, MCOs tend to favor drug therapy over psychotherapy (McFarland, 1994). More MCOs will pay for pharmacotherapy even when the medications are more expensive than sessions of therapy with a mental health professional (Sturm & Wells, 1995). The type of analysis done by these providers omits half of the equation, as the combination of drugs and psychotherapy has been shown to be most effective in the treatment of depression, as well as in other disorders that tend to disproportionately affect women such as eating disorders, panic attacks, and obsessive-compulsive disorders (Gonen, 1997).

Outpatient mental health care is the less expensive alternative to inpatient treatment (Miller, 1996). However, there continue to be insurance company financial incentives that favor inpatient care even when it is less efficient than outpatient treatment (Ackley, 1993; Kiesler, 1992; Lowman, 1991). Considerable research indicates that outpatient treatment is, in many cases, the treatment of choice (Kiesler, 1992) and would therefore be the logical choice for higher rates of coverage. However, 83.8% of HMOs offer the option of zero copayment for inpatient mental health care, while only 26.6% offer the same plan for outpatient mental heath care (Group Health Association of America, 1995).

When outpatient psychotherapy is allowed by a managed care organization, providers are required to minimize costs by greatly limiting the number of sessions available. Miller (1996) states that a reduction in the average length of treatment to the 2.5 to 6.6 session range, which managed care groups encourage, requires therapy much shorter than that which treatment reviews have traditionally cited as brief therapy. Treatment of this length, Miller (1996) explains, should be referred to as "ultrabrief therapy." However, there are no controlled studies of ultrabrief therapy.

The Follette and Cummings (1967) study frequently cited by MCOs as justifying the use of ultrabrief therapy is, to quote Miller (1996), "very weak evidence for the effectiveness of ultrabrief therapy." In addition, Mumford, Schlesinger, Glass, Patrick and Cuerdon's (1984) study, another examination of the effectiveness of very small "doses" of psychotherapy, found no effect for less than four psychotherapy visits, strongly contradicting the assumptions of MCOs that minimal therapy is adequate therapy.

The managed care industry has responded to these criticisms, that the industry overly emphasizes drug therapy and offers too few sessions, with outcome data to prove the effectiveness of their treatments. Outcome data that adequately assesses the effectiveness of therapy is so complex as to have required meta-analyses (Lipsey & Wilson, 1993). Instead, most MCOs want customer satisfaction data (Miller,

1996). Companies such as Press/Ganney Associates (1998) market such outcome questionnaires. Questions include: convenience of available appointment times, helpfulness of office staff, privacy of the treatment area, etc. These types of customer satisfaction reports are particularly troublesome because they do not objectively rate the effectiveness of treatment. In fact, these types of ratings may not rate the treatment at all and when they do are prone to inflation due to such variables as pleasing the therapist and trying to give the impression of being a healthy and successful client. These inflated statistics may falsely give the impression of effective therapy when in fact it has not taken place (Miller, 1996).

WOMEN, MANAGED CARE AND MENTAL HEALTH

Factory labor, "pink collar" workers, and women who work inside the home are particularly affected by the onset of managed care in mental health. Large industrial companies often contract with "super-groups" for exclusive mental health coverage. In other words, all of their employees, in order to use their insurance benefits, must go to the same practice. These practices are typically very large and are frequently owned by health care conglomerates. The emphasis within these practices is, as previously outlined, on rapidity of care and cost containment. "Pink collar" workers, women who work in the "women's work" fields, often do not have insurance provided to them at all. In fact, a study by the Commonwealth Fund (1995) found that fifteen percent of all women ages 18 to 64 had no health insurance. For those that do receive insurance through their employment, mental health benefits are often very limited and associated with managed care. These women are often unable to pay for private psychotherapy when the managed care benefits are exhausted. Community mental health may provide an important resource. These centers, which although sometimes quite high in quality, are often inconsistent in the training and quality of staff as well as being subject to the whims of public funding. In addition, many of these centers are themselves becoming affiliated with MCOs. Finally, women who do not work outside the home who either have no insurance or receive Medicare or Medicaid are further restricted in their mental health choices as managed care enrolls increasing numbers of these programs' participants.

Women, as the primary consumers of outpatient mental health care,

are differentially affected by these developments (Davis, 1996). Over-all rates of mental illness are approximately the same for men and women, but women suffer more from depression and anxiety disorders while men experience higher rates of substance and alcohol abuse and personality disorders (Commonwealth Fund, 1995). Major depression is the most common severe mental disorder among women, currently affecting approximately 7 million American women.

Despite the high morbidity associated with depression and anxiety, the majority of episodes go undetected and therefore untreated, in large part because our health care system is based on a biomedical, treatment only as "medically necessary," model. One study of 1,000 patients with depression found that those enrolled in managed care were properly diagnosed only 40 percent of the time (Gonen, 1997). In part because of the traditional division between physical and mental health and the stigma associated with mental health treatment, the majority of mental disorders are diagnosed and treated within the general medical sector (McFarland, 1994) which can compromise the quality of care received (Sturm & Wells, 1995).

Many women do not receive necessary care at all. Passive attitudes, concerns about stigma, and low self-esteem lead some women to avoid mental health treatment altogether. Obligations to children, family, and work create real constraints on seeking this type of care. These barriers are further complicated by the absence of health insurance or exclusions and limits on mental health services (Davis, 1996).

A paper commissioned by the Commonwealth Fund (1995) con-cluded that much of the care women receive for psychological prob-lems takes place outside the professional mental health system, much of it being provided by general health physicians. Unfortunately, pri-mary care providers have not been well trained to accept this role and this may pose a problem as managed care further expands the role of the primary care physician.

As managed care has changed the way that health care, and espe-cially mental health care, is paid for and allocated, so must managed care change to serve adequately its enrollees, especially women. These changes must include parity of payment for mental health care, length and type of treatment at the discretion of the client and provider, and appropriate training in women's mental health issues for all involved healthcare providers. Managed care cannot be allowed to remain a second tier of coverage. In the same way that psychotherapy empowers those left out of the economic system, so must psychotherapy practitioners empower themselves to benefit from and perhaps control the future of managed behavioral health care.

REFERENCES

Ackley, D.C. (1993). Employee health insurance benefits: A comparison of managed care with traditional mental health care: Costs and results. *The Independent Practitioner, 13*, 49-53.

American Association of Health Plans. (1996). *Demographic characteristics of health plan enrollees.* Washington, DC: Author.

Commonwealth Fund. (1995). *Women and mental health: Issues for health reform.* [on-line], Available: *www.cmwf.org*

Davis, K. (1996). *The bottom line–HMOs and mental health.* Briefing note. The Commonwealth Fund, October.

Follette, W.T., & Cummings, N.A. (1967). Psychiatric services and medical utilization in a prepaid health plan setting. *Medical Care, 5*, 25-35.

Gonen, J.S. (1997). Managed care and women's mental health: A focus on depression. *Insights–Jacobs Institute of Women's Health* [on-line], 5. Available: www.jiwh.org/insights/dec97no5.htm

Group Health Association of America. (1995). Coverage of selected benefits by HMOs with point of service products, 1995. *GHAA's Annual HMO Industry Survey.*

Health Care Financing Administration. (1998). *Carrier specific file, physician fee schedule payment amount* [on-line]. Available: www.HCFA.gov/stats/98carr.htm

Kaiser Family Foundation. (January, 1998). *Kaiser/Harvard national survey of Americans' views on consumer protection in managed care* [on-line]. Available: http: *www.kff.org/archive/health_policy/general/bill/bill_rep.html*

Kiesler, C.A. (1992). U.S. mental health policies: Doomed to fail. *American Psychologist, 47*, 1077-1082.

Lipsey, M.W., & Wilson, D.B. (1993). The efficacy of psychological, educational, and behavioral treatment. *American Psychologist, 48*, 1181-1209.

Lowman, R.L. (1991). Mental health claims experience: Analysis and benefit redesign. *Professional Psychology: Research and Practice, 22*, 36-44.

McFarland, B.H. (1994). Cost-effectiveness considerations for managed care systems: Treating depression in primary care. *American Journal of Medicine, 97 (supplement).* 6a-47s.

Miller, I.J. (1996). Managed care is harmful to outpatient mental health services: A call for accountability. *Professional Psychology: Research and Practice, 27*, 349-363.

Mumford, E., Schlesinger, H.J., Glass, G.V., Patrick, C., & Cuerdon, T. (1984). A new look at evidence about reduced cost of medical utilization following mental health treatment. *The American Journal of Psychiatry, 141*, 1145-1158.

National Center for Health Statistics. (1997) National ambulatory medical care survey: 1996 summary. *Advance Data–Centers for Disease Control and Prevention, 295*, 1-28.

National Research Corporation. (1996). *Health care market guide survey.* Washington, DC: Author.

Press-Ganey. (1998). *Outpatient mental health questionnaire* [on-line]. Available: www.pressganey.com/products/opmh.htm

Sturm, R. & Wells, K. (1995). How can care for depression become more cost-effective? *Journal of the American Medical Association, 237*, 1.

The Function
of the Frame and the Role of Fee
in the Therapeutic Situation

Stephanie Buck

SUMMARY. Money is a concrete representation of energy. As such, it is a primary vehicle for the exchange of individual and collective energy in consumer-based societies. It is also an archetypal symbol of power that signifies much about the person who possesses it and how she or he uses power in relationship to self and others. Because money is the symbolic carrier of energy and power, it is also a representation of the therapy itself. Therefore, all aspects of fee such as what form it takes, how much, who pays and when to pay are all of the utmost importance. The manner in which the therapist addresses the issue of fee as well as the other ground rules and her ability to both secure and maintain the therapeutic frame at the initial session and later will set the course of therapy. *[Article copies available for a fee from The Haworth Document Delivery Service: 1-800-342-9678. E-mail address: getinfo@haworthpressinc.com <Website: http://www.haworthpressinc.com>]*

KEYWORDS. Therapeutic frame, bipersonal field, archetypal symbol

THE FRAME AS CONTAINER

The success or failure of psychotherapy is dependent upon the ability of the therapist to create and maintain a secure frame in which

Stephanie Buck, MA, a licensed psychotherapist practicing in central Vermont, is currently working on her doctorate in Analytical Psychology at The Union Institute.

Address correspondence to: Stephanie Buck, 2005 Bull Run Road, Northfield, VT 05663.

[Haworth co-indexing entry note]: "The Function of the Frame and the Role of Fee in the Therapeutic Situation." Buck, Stephanie. Co-published simultaneously in *Women & Therapy* (The Haworth Press, Inc.) Vol. 22, No. 3, 1999, pp. 37-50; and: *For Love or Money: The Fee in Feminist Therapy* (eds: Marcia Hill, and Ellyn Kaschak) The Haworth Press, Inc., 1999, pp. 37-50. Single or multiple copies of this article are available for a fee from The Haworth Document Delivery Service [1-800-342-9678, 9:00 a.m. - 5:00 p.m. (EST). E-mail address: getinfo@haworthpressinc.com].

the work of therapy can develop. Setting, time, session length, duration of treatment, fee, confidentiality and the "rules" of client participation and therapist intervention are the components that constitute the frame of therapy (Langs, 1985). Just like "the frame of a painting [that sets] off the reality inside from the reality outside" (Milner, cited in Langs & Stone, 1980, p. 45), and holds the painting securely in place, the therapeutic frame holds both the client and the therapist within an ordered and secure setting. The boundaries created by the institution of these conditions of therapy and their management set the therapy and the dyadic relationship of therapist and client apart from the reality of the world thereby creating a maternal holding environment wherein the work of therapy can safely unfold (Winnicott, 1990). In this way, the therapeutic relationship in its dependency on a secure frame for the establishment of a solid foundation for the work that ensues is similar to the mother-child relationship which develops within the maternal matrix of a secure holding environment (Conforti, 1988). It is the mother's capacity for *reverie* [italics added] with her infant–the extent to which she is able to contain the infant's affective states and allow the infant's reintrojection of the maternal hold–that will help determine the course of the infant's development; safely held within the embrace of the maternal container, the infant comes to know itself (Bion, 1993). In a similar way, the client comes to know himself or herself through the therapeutic relationship that develops within the container of a secure frame. Conforti (1988) writes:

> The importance of the quality of the maternal hold and its effects on the child highlight the important effect that the psychological well-being of the analyst and his ability to maintain the analytic structure has on the client and the outcome of analysis. (introduction)

As the very real foundation for the work of therapy, the frame nurtures the bipersonal field of client-therapist interactions "based on the respective intrapsychic needs and sets, evocations and reactions–adaptive responses–of each party" (Langs, 1990, p. 292). The primary function of the frame, then, is that of a container, which Jung (1944/1993) described as the *vas bene clausum*, the well-sealed vessel:

> that protect[s] what is within from the intrusion and admixture of what is without. . . . [so that there] is the active evocation of inner

images . . . an authentic feat of thought or ideation, which . . . does not, that is to say, just play with its objects, but tries to grasp the inner facts and portray them in images true to their nature. (p. 167)

Of these images, Jung (1965) writes:

We allow the images to rise up, and maybe we wonder about them, but that is all. We do not take the trouble to understand them, let alone draw ethical conclusions from them. This stopping-short conjures up the negative effects of the unconscious . . . . The images of the unconscious place a great responsibility upon a man. Failure to understand them, or a shirking of ethical responsibility, deprives him of his wholeness and imposes a painful fragmentation on his life. (p. 192, 193)

Langs (1985) calls these images "transformed images," products of primary-process narratives and the visual imagery of layered meanings. Unlike secondary-process thinking, which "is attuned to the external world" and is "logical, sequential and confined to manifest thinking," primary-process thinking "is fluid and unconcerned with objective reality or sequential time. It readily shifts about without linear focus, and uses a set of specific and unique mechanisms in its operation" (p. 3). In the depth model, "the patient's unconscious leads, and is alone to be pursued" (Winnicott, 1990, p. 416). The well-structured and managed frame supports this intrapsychic journey.

The frame sets the therapy apart from ordinary life and holds the client securely and safely within the constancy of its sphere so that another level of reality–that of the client's inner psychic world of *imago* (his or her subjective experience combined with archetypal images), accessed through transformed images–is enabled to emerge and take shape. For this to occur, the frame conditions or ground rules that form the boundaries of the therapy must be maintained and managed by the therapist; in this respect, the therapeutic frame is a living and active entity. Because the work of therapy is contingent upon the working alliance created at the outset of treatment between client and therapist, the frame structures a bipersonal field of interaction. Regarded in this way, a primary function of the depth model of psychotherapy can no longer be understood as the client's working through of transference issues as if his or her experiences in relationship to the therapist were solely self-referential as interpreted in the classic transference-countertransference model. Within the bipersonal field of the therapy, the therapist's as well as the client's issues are constellated within the relationship.

Feminist psychotherapy, in particular, rejects psychoanalysis's error-laden construction of transference and countertransference within the therapy relationship where the "individual is separated out from context [and] studied as a self-contained being" (Jordan, Kaplan, Miller, Stiver & Surrey, 1991, p. 81) by the therapist who acts as a blank-screen upon which the client's psychic conflicts are projected. Instead, feminist psychotherapy, because it is rooted in the ground of women's experience, considers all that shapes women's lives to be of the utmost importance to the work of therapy. The feminist approach, represented by the ongoing work of The Stone Center, is concerned with women's "growth through and toward relationship," which Jordan et al. term "relational mutuality." Jordan writes:

> The traditional therapy model of looking at intrapsychic factors, the "I," the one-person system provides important insights, but acknowledging the importance of the relationship, context, the quality of interaction and the deeply intersubjective nature of human lives greatly expands our understanding of the people with whom we work. (Jordan et al., 1991, pp. 81, 82)

Feminist psychodynamic psychotherapy and analytical psychotherapy share a similar attitude regarding the importance of a therapist's genuineness within the therapy relationship. What Jordan calls "relational mutuality," Jung might have labeled the "human factor" (Fordham, 1978). In both instances, the emphasis is on the potential curative powers of the relational process itself. When all the ground rules of the therapy hour are instituted and maintained during the course of treatment, the protective space that is created within its bounds contains this relationship and supports the ever-deepening work of the therapy. Thus, the client-therapist relationship that gradually develops within this container of the frame *is* representative of the work since all that the client struggles with will play out in the present moment of the therapeutic relationship. The therapist's capacity for containing and working with client material, in addition to containing his or her own issues, will be evidenced by how well the therapist creates and cares for the structure of the therapy (Conforti, 1988).

A secure frame of static ground rules and set limits provides the therapist with the necessary context for accurately identifying the dynamic interplay occurring between himself or herself and the client. For example, if the therapist has not sufficiently addressed his or her own issues regarding mortality, which Langs calls existential death anxiety (Langs, 1997), he or she will not be able to contain that of the client, and each will act and react out of a *manic defense*. Of the manic defense, Winnicott (1992) states that "the manic defense is the employment of almost any opposites in the reassurance against death, chaos and mystery" (p. 132). This defensive structure closes off the client (and the therapist who engages with it) from internal psychic reality (Conforti, 1988). The result is a manifest level of communication, i.e., secondary-process thinking, where no real work can happen since, within the model of depth therapy, "unconscious factors contribute to surface madness" (Langs, 1985, p. 3) and must be addressed for change to occur.

When the therapist is unable to hold the client appropriately, manifested by the therapist's beginning therapy early or late, going over the allotted time for the session, setting an inappropriate fee or no fee at all, self-disclosure or breaking confidentiality by allowing a third party into the privacy of the session, etc., the frame cannot be closed, the healing work cannot proceed and the therapy becomes "stuck." What results is a "therapeutic misalliance" rather than the necessary working alliance between therapist and client. According to Langs (1990), "there are inherent needs in both patient and analyst to both create and resolve therapeutic misalliances in every analytic and psychotherapeutic situation, and that [*sic*] the recognition, analysis, and modification of these propensities and actualities is a first-order therapeutic task" (p. 291). In other words, the natural state of therapy includes both adherence to frame structure and attempts to deviate from it on the part of both client and therapist. The therapist's task is to understand the drama being enacted *within* the therapy relationship indicated by what Langs calls the "adaptive context" (the frame condition that is being compromised, for example) and to intervene based on the information presenting itself. A secure frame (recall Jung's *vas bene clausum*) provides a stable environment for the developing work; it enables the therapist more accurately to assess client material within the bipersonal field because disruptions to the conditions of therapy are placed within the context of the client-therapist relationship and serve as a reference point for the work.

Conforti presents another way to understand the phenomenon of the therapeutic alliance/misalliance within the container of the therapeutic frame. He posits that there is an archetypal configuration to the client and therapist coupling. Rather than being a "misalliance" as Langs suggests, this archetypal coupling of client and therapist results from the "entrainment" of the archetypal field of each so that a third field–the therapy relationship–is created and enacted within the therapy. Conforti (1997) writes:

> I realized there was a symmetry or synchronization of psyches going on in the therapeutic situation, whereby both client and therapist were entrained around some specific archetypal dynamic. Entraining has to do with the spontaneous synchronization of previously disparate parts of a system. This is dramatically represented by the collective force of a squadron marching in unison across a bridge. The force is tremendous, so much so that if the soldiers do not break step, and break this synchronized movement, they could collapse a bridge. (p. 4)

The entrainment of each party to this dominant archetype that energizes the therapy field will be suggested both by client attempts to modify the frame and by the therapist's response or reaction to these frame demands. In both situations, what is manifested in thought, affect and behavior will indicate the archetypal dominant of the therapy relationship and the way in which the client and therapist are entrained within the archetypal matrix of the therapy field. The therapist's identification and interpretation of this archetypal dynamic in the relationship and its amplification is the work of therapy so that, where necessary, the client's inappropriate ego alignment is shifted to a more appropriate, healthy alignment to the archetype.

Conforti (1996) furthers our understanding of the archetype's influence and significance with his conceptualization of therapy as an archetypal field wherein the archetypal processes of both the client and therapist are interactionally engaged to a specific purpose that can be identified through its representation in space and time. Jung's (1989) explanation of archetypes as:

forms or images of a collective nature which occur practically all over the earth as constituents of myths and at the same time as autochthonous, individual products of unconscious origin. The[se] archetypal motifs presumably derive from patterns of the human mind that are transmitted not only by tradition and migration but also heredity. The later hypothesis is indispensable, since even complicated archetypal images can be reproduced spontaneously without there being any possibility of direct tradition (p. 50)

does not address the "complexing" aspect of the archetype, the power of an archetype to attract and pull a therapist and client, for example, into an entrainment around a certain idea, image, etc. that then takes on a dynamic life of its own separate from ego consciousness. Conforti's hypothesis of archetypal entrainment within a field does address the complexing aspect and will be explored shortly around the issue of the therapy fee and the money complex.

All of the framing elements of the therapy–setting, session length and duration, fee, confidentiality, client free association and therapist interventions–are necessary to contain securely the work that develops within the archetypal field of the therapeutic relationship. These ground rules are, in fact, dependent upon one another since the therapist cannot address one frame condition without touching upon the others in some way (Langs, 1985). Recall the analogy of the picture frame used at the beginning of this paper: the function of the frame is to separate the internal from the external and to secure in place that which the frame's sides surround. If one or more sides of the frame is missing, i.e., if one or more ground rules of the therapy is absent, broken or modified, there is insufficient separation. These "cracks in the frame" (Margolies, 1990) or frame deviations (Langs, 1985), prevent closure of the frame so that the therapy situation is not secure for the vital intrapsychic work of dynamic psychotherapy.

THE DYNAMIC ROLE OF FEE

Although all of the conditions of therapy are needed to frame and ground the work, one especially–the therapy fee–is of particular concern because of what it represents: the therapist-client commitment to the work of therapy. As a tangible symbol of the ever-unfolding process of individuation (movement toward psychic wholeness and balance), the fee drives the therapy. That the fee should be such a powerful and energetic carrier of the work is not surprising since, according to Lockhart, Hillman, Vasavada, Perry, Covitz and Guggenbuhl-Craig (1982), "money is the most powerful, practical and experienced form of transformation" (p. 14). In the form of coinage, money is in fact a symbol of the Self (Lockhart et al.). Dynamic psychotherapy, particularly analytical or Jungian psychotherapy, ultimately is concerned with the client's transformation from disease to harmony with Self, which both regulates the individual's psyche and represents the totality of his or her personality. Jung (1965) writes:

> The self is not only the centre but also the whole circumference which embraces both conscious and unconscious; it is the centre of this totality, just as the ego is the centre of consciousness. . . . the self is our life's goal, for it is the completest expression of that fateful combination we call individuality. (p. 398)

With this understanding of the essential significance of the therapy fee–fee in the form of money as an archetypal symbol of the client's psychic potentiality–all aspects of fee such as what form it takes, how much, is it set or flexible, who pays and when to pay are all of the utmost importance and need to be considered by the therapist when setting the client's fee. Unfortunately, the energetic reality of the fee as the representation of the dynamic principle of psyche at work in the therapy is usually not given its due, even by some analysts. Thus, one considers that "Soul Work is not a professional work for money . . . Give me happily and freely whatever you can conveniently and without restraint," while another "prefer[s] not to think about money . . . allowing people to run up inordinate bills that sometimes go unpaid" (Lockhart et al., 1982, pp. 47, 57). Even Jung was criticized by his fellow analysts for undercharging his patients, thereby diminishing, they believed, their practices (Lockhart et al., p. 57).

Other fee practices, such as barter, gifts, loans and free therapy are not uncommon especially for those therapists who practice within the socio-political perspective of the feminist model (Margolies, 1990). Feminist therapy has provided a very necessary framework from which to understand oppression and the systemic inter-workings of power and control dynamics. Its strength lies in its social conscience where the classic developmental theories and clinical practices are tested against the reality of women's lives and found wanting. Within feminist therapy, certain frame components such as fee and disclosure are emblematic of the feminist relational model where "the personal is political." The truth of women's economic oppression and the many ways in which women's voices have been silenced within the masculinist paradigm must be addressed in order for these and other injustices to be rectified. The feminist therapy model provides one very important avenue through which clients can approach these and other issues from the context of their lives and that of society.

Analytical psychology, with its emphasis on the guiding influence of archetypes in the lives of individuals and the collective, moves beyond and below the reality of everyday concerns to the realm of the Self. It is here, at the core of psyche, where first order change occurs; symbols, as expressions of the archetype, mark the client's way toward individuation. In this way, by providing the individual and the collective with a "path" to wholeness, feminist therapy and analytical psychotherapy are complementary.

Divergence in therapists' attitudes and practices regarding fee management is not due solely to differences in theoretical orientation, however, although the different psychotherapeutic understandings that therapists hold obviously do shape the way in which they work with clients around fee as well as around the other frame issues. The difference in belief and approach to fee that therapists (and clients) hold is rooted in the quality of money itself and in the fact that "everyone has a money complex, and the way each person relates to money can have a profound effect on other areas of his life" (Lockhart et al., 1982, p. 63). Hillman (in Lockhart et al., 1982) captures the emotional charge of the complex and the oppositional pull that it energizes between one's unassimilated affects concerning some *thing* and one's habitual conscious attitude toward it, for example, money, when he writes that "the fear of money and the importance of money in some persons may be more psychologically devastating, and therefore rewarding, than sexual fears and impotence" (p. 41). When therapists deny this reality of money by only considering its manifest significance, i.e., the economic cost to themselves and their clients, the deep work of therapy is diminished. Reduced fees, exorbitant fees, no fees, barter, gifts and loans are all aspects of the archetypal symbol of money, but because each transaction represents a unique relationship toward the central archetype of Self, each carries a different energetic charge that will have an impact on the generative effect of therapy.

Covitz (in Lockhart et al., 1982) points out that the ancient Greeks "correlated the absence of money with the disease process and its presence with the cure" (p. 63); in the ancient world, bodily sickness and psychic distress were an inseparable unity (Meier, 1989). Because all that we are and all that is potential within us, both as individuals and as a culture, is archetypally based and because the "life of the past [that] still exists in us with the life of the present" (Jung, 1951/1990, p. 157), other, older attitudes influence us today. Thus, when therapists do not attend to the archetypal significance of fee in their frame decisions, the "soul" consequences to their clients are serious and what is enacted in order to be helpful/supportive is in reality harmful.

Money is at one and the same time abstract and concrete. In a very real sense, money has two sides–think of two sides of the coin–the spiritual and the secular (Lockhart et al., 1982). The essence of money, that which is most "real" about it, is its energy (one side of the coin). Energy, the dynamic property of money, is revealed by the power to purchase which is conferred upon the holder (the other side of the coin). In Western culture, money's capacity to transform the potentialities of life (abstract energy) into realities (concrete form) identifies it as the archetypal expression of the Self–the purposeful center of psyche–and the therapy fee as the ideal carrier of the transformative work of therapy. Money, in effect, symbolizes everything so that "nothing else achieves this range of transformational possibility in actuality or fantasy" (Lockhart et al., p. 15). Because money stands for what is potential in all of us, it is an archetypal symbol around which all of our unresolved issues concerning self constellate; it is but one of the many *complexes,* the emotional "hot spots," that dwell within our psyche and form the basis of who we are. How we engage with this manifestation of the archetype and navigate between its poles, i.e., poverty and luxury, generosity and miserliness, joy and fear (Lockhart et al., 1982), says much about our relation to psyche and the way in which we enact this relationship in the outer world.

The money complex is one of the innumerable complexes around which the therapist and client become *entrained* within the archetypal third field of the therapy relationship. It is activated and spins its mindless course when therapist and client alike collude around fee and other frame issues. For example: the therapist sets an inappropriately low fee, reduces the set fee or waives the fee altogether in *reaction* (unconscious action) to the client's request rather than making an interpretation based on an understanding of the psychodynamics currently being enacted within the field and then proceeding from there. When the therapist reacts to the client's reaction to frame conditions (secure frame dread), both are aligned in a manic defense (recall both Winnicott's and Langs' understanding of this frame-related psychic position addressed earlier in the paper) and closed off to the present creative moment of therapy. When the therapist intervenes with an interpretation of the psychodynamic event, he or she is "holding" the client in a healing way because he or she is *responding* (conscious action) to the client's painful intrapsychic drama that is presently being enacted in the request for frame deviance. There will invariably be instances within the therapy relationship when the therapist will need to be flexible around certain frame related issues (for example, cancelled sessions or planned absences which are adaptations to the existing frame and therefore, deviations to the frame). Any change to the conditions of therapy by either party, whether driven by necessity or otherwise, will impact the work and is representative of the intrapsychic issue being worked over by the client in the therapy relationship.

Therapy is a journey of transformation that the client embarks on with the support of the therapist. The universal stories of transformation, such as myths of the hero's quest epitomized by Galahad's search for the Holy Grail and myths of the cycle of renewal poignantly represented by Demeter's search for the abducted Persephone, are archetypal templates that each particular client's path follows: night-sea-journey, the dark night of the soul and descent into the underworld are the varied ways used to describe this voyage of discovery. As these names imply, the client's movement towards wholeness is perilous and, just as in the tranformation myths, always demands both a dying to the old self so that a new one can emerge, and a sacrifice.

In therapy, the fee is the sacrifice that generates the work and moves the client along the way as he or she navigates the shores of consciousness and the deep waters of the unconscious psyche. In the myth of Hades, Charon, the boatman, ferried the dead across the sacred river Styx which divided the land of the living from the realm of the dead, the underworld. For this service, he exacted a toll of his passengers, the payment of a coin that each spirit carried in his hand, between his lips or on his eyelid (Morford & Lenardon, 1977; Walker, 1996). Those who could not pay were left ashore (Morford & Lenardon,

1977). Like Charon, who carries his charges from one realm to the next for the set payment of a coin, "analyst [or therapist] carries the problems of the patient for a fee" (Lockhart et al., 1982, p. 79). The exchange binds the relationship and assures a safe crossing. The coin, as the symbol of potentiality made manifest (the conversion of energy into matter) represents the commitment of each party to meet the responsibilities of their respective tasks: the client to metaphorically walk the difficult path to Self and the therapist to support and guide the way. Training, skill, time and self are all the resources that the therapist commits in the service of the client. Covitz (in Lockhart et al., 1982) uses an analogy between the following service notice and the therapist-client exchange in order to highlight the important connection between fee and therapy:

> Never buy what you do not want because it is cheap; it will be dear to you. I have at home an ad for paint which states: "Don't blame the painter. If the painter has to use cheap materials to meet your price ideas, you've no kick coming if the job doesn't last. Pay a fair price for good honest varnish, enamel and paint." (p. 79)

CONCLUSION

The therapy fee is perhaps the most complex and least understood of the various frame components. It encompasses not only the obvious mechanics of how much, who pays and when, but also is tied to the other frame issues such as confidentiality (third party payments) and payment for client absences. Most importantly, the fee is the expression of the central archetype of Self that purposefully moves all of us toward individuation, a lifelong process of integration to wholeness. Because fee symbolizes this generative principle of psyche, it must be respected for its power and treated accordingly in the therapy. Other aspects of fee need to be addressed as well; as technology changes the form that money takes and its transport, i.e., charge cards and automatic deposit, the method of exchange between client and therapist changes. What are the resulting energetic consequences to these economic advances which bypass the life-affirming process of energy conversion into matter and represented by paper money, coin and check? Because fee symbolizes the transformative work of psyche in the therapy process, this shift in exchange matters. Concerning money, the tangible expression of human energy and potential, Doty (1978) writes that:

> throughout the many centuries of their existence, coins have been intimately connected to the larger story of human history, joined so closely, in fact, that much of the story of man's development–the rise and fall of great empires, the flowerings and eclipses of artistic inspiration–may be traced and chronicled through coins. For no other product of the human mind, over so many centuries, can this claim be made. (p. 8)

How the therapist deals with the question of fee will depend not only on his or her theoretical understanding of the role of money in the therapy relationship, but also, and more importantly, on his or her personal relationship to money, the archetypal symbol of his or her relationship to Self.

REFERENCES

Bion, W.R. (1993). *Second thoughts: Selected papers on psycho-analysis.* Northvale, NJ: Jason Aronson.

Conforti, M. (1988). *Unconscious dynamics of the initial interview situation: Phenomenological study of patients' unconscious response to the conditions of treatment.* Unpublished doctoral dissertation, The Union Institute, Cincinnati, OH.

Conforti, M. (1996). On archetypal fields. *The Round Table Review: Of contemporary contributions to Jungian psychology, 4,* 1-8.

Conforti, M. (1997). A symmetry of psyches: Experiences of the confluence of the new sciences & Jungian psychology. *The Round Table Review: Of contemporary contributions to Jungian psychology, 5,* 4-10.

Doty, R. (1978). *Money and the world.* New York: Grosset & Dunlap.

Fordham, M. (1978). Some idiosyncratic behaviour of therapists. *Journal of Analytical Psychology, 23*(2), 122-134.

Jordan, V.J., Kaplan, A.G., Miller, J.B., Stiver, I.P. & Surrey, J.L. (1991). *Women's growth in connection: Writings from The Stone Center.* New York: The Guilford Press.

Jung, C.G. (1965). *Memories, dreams, reflections.* (R. & C. Winston, Trans.). New York: Vintage Books.

Jung, C. G. (1989). Psychology and religion. In *Collected works* (2nd ed.) (Vol. 11, pp. 3-105). Princeton, NJ: Princeton University Press.

Jung, C.G. (1990). The psychology of the child archetype. (R.F.C. Hull, Trans.). In *Collected works* (Vol. 9i, pp. 151-181). Princeton, NJ: Princeton University Press. (Original work published 1951).

Jung, C.G. (1993). The symbolism of the mandala. (R.F.C. Hull, Trans.). In *Collected works* (Rev. ed.) (Vol. 12, pp. 95-223). Princeton, NJ: Princeton University Press. (Original work published 1944).

Langs, R. (1985). *Workbooks for psychotherapists: Understanding unconscious communication* (Vol. 1). Emerson, NJ: NewConcept Press.

Langs, R. (1990). Therapeutic misalliances. In R. Langs (Ed.), *Classics in psychoanalytic technique* (Rev. ed.) (pp. 291-306). Northvale, NJ: Jason Aronson.

Langs, R. (1997). *Death anxiety and clinical practice.* London: Karnac Books.

Langs, R., & Stone, L. (1980). *The therapeutic experience and its setting: A clinical dialogue.* New York: Jason Aronson.

Lockhart, R., Hillman, J., Vasavada, A., Perry, J.W., Covitz, J.I., & Guggenbuhl-Craig, A. (1982). *Soul and money.* Dallas: Spring Publications.

Margolies, L. (1990). Cracks in the frame: Feminism and the boundaries of therapy. *Women & Therapy, 9*(4), 19-31.

Meier, C.A. (1989). *Healing dream and ritual.* Einsiedein, Switzerland: Daimon Verlag.

Morford, M. & Lenardon, R. (1977). *Classical mythology.* (2nd ed.). New York: Longman.

Walker, B. (1996). *The women's encyclopedia of myths and secrets.* Edison, NJ: Castle Books.

Winnicott, D.W. (1992). The manic defence. In D.W. Winnicott (Ed.), *Through pediatrics to psycho-analysis: Collected papers.* (pp. 129-144). New York: Brunner/Mazel.

Winnicott, D.W. (1990). On transference. In R. Langs (Ed.), *Classics in psycho-analytic technique.* (pp. 415-418). Northvale, NJ: Jason Aronson.

Payment for Missed Sessions: Policy, Countertransference and Other Challenges

Evelyn Sommers

SUMMARY. The policy of requiring payment for sessions canceled without adequate notice can result in dilemmas that many therapists wish to avoid. In this exploration, sound clinical reasons for enforcing payment under such circumstances, including the acquisition of therapeutic insight and modeled assertive behaviors, are discussed using case examples incorporating an examination of countertransference. One exception to this position, in which flexibility is recommended, is also described. The discussion removes the issue of payment from the concrete domain of money for service by conceptualizing the scheduled appointment as a promise between therapist and client, late cancellations as unconscious challenges to the promise, and enforcement of payment as a means of protecting the promise. Therapists are encouraged to examine feelings that might interfere with their ability to follow through on their own payment policies. *[Article copies available for a fee from The Haworth Document Delivery Service: 1-800-342-9678. E-mail address: getinfo@haworthpressinc.com <Website: http://www.haworthpressinc.com>]*

KEYWORDS. Payment policy, cancellations, feminist, modeling, countertransference

Evelyn Sommers, PhD, is a psychologist in practice as a psychotherapist in Toronto, Canada.

Address correspondence to: Evelyn Sommers, 683 Annette Street, Toronto, Ontario, Canada, M6S 2C9.

[Haworth co-indexing entry note]: "Payment for Missed Sessions: Policy, Countertransference and Other Challenges." Sommers, Evelyn. Co-published simultaneously in *Women & Therapy* (The Haworth Press, Inc.) Vol. 22, No. 3, 1999, pp. 51-68; and: *For Love or Money: The Fee in Feminist Therapy* (eds: Marcia Hill, and Ellyn Kaschak) The Haworth Press, Inc., 1999, pp. 51-68. Single or multiple copies of this article are available for a fee from The Haworth Document Delivery Service [1-800-342-9678, 9:00 a.m. - 5:00 p.m. (EST). E-mail address: getinfo@haworthpressinc.com].

51

Like many practitioners in helping professions, I have a policy of charging the full fee for missed sessions unless I am given a specified notice of cancellation. Clients are informed of the policy during the first telephone contact and the first session. The only exceptions are for cancellations due to sudden illness, accident, or life and death situations. From time to time I have been confronted with challenges to the policy, leading me to reflect on the implications of creating and "enforcing" a policy of payment. In one instance, a client left a message on the morning of her weekly appointment to say that her daughter was arriving that day for a brief visit, so she would not be attending her session. The next week the client failed to mention her obligation to pay for the canceled session. I then had to choose a course of action taking into account boundary issues, clinical judgments, and my feelings about setting and standing firm on limits, all within the highly emotional domain of fee for service. Many therapists react to such dilemmas with a wish to avoid them, a feeling I have shared. Indeed, this writing was inspired by my struggles with payment issues, as well as by clients who have commented on the value of the difficult but rewarding "enforcement" sessions that have occurred as an outcome of their challenges to my policy.

Discussions with colleagues and articles by authors such as Michele Bograd (1991) have underscored the struggles with payment issues that are common to many practitioners, especially those who attempt to work collaboratively with their clients or are concerned about issues of fee setting related to the ability of clients to pay, along with consideration of their own needs. Dealing with the exchange of money for counseling and psychotherapy is often considered an annoying and distasteful task, and asking for payment when a session has not occurred presents special difficulties for those who think of themselves as helpers. Yet psychologists and counselors providing services in private practice must address, directly or indirectly, the issue of payment with each client who engages their services. Fees must be named; invoices must be presented and paid; insurance forms must be signed for payment; availability and limits of benefits, billing practices and other related matters must be discussed. Frequently these discussions of payment are viewed as an imposition on the therapy relationship, stealing time away from the "real" stuff of psychotherapy and engendering a possible threat to the process. However, money is a fundamental, practical, and emotional factor in our lives and it is important for the upkeep and well-being of us all. Therefore, money in some ways levels the intersubjective field between client and therapist as well as introducing an additional level of complexity. Thus, the process of exchanging money for service presents a rich source of psychological material and challenges for the therapist and client to address in the here-and-now of the therapeutic relationship. Many concerns related to this topic are discussed elsewhere (e.g., Krueger, 1986) such as determinants of policy and the fact that a policy which allows for exceptions to payment places the therapist in the uncomfortable position of having to judge the merit of absences. My focus in this discussion is on the issues and effects arising when a policy requiring payment for missed sessions after the requested notice is not given was enforced. I also describe a situation in which it was therapeutically helpful to be flexible when a client protested paying for missed sessions. Underlying the different decisions was my wish to establish and maintain trust by creating a secure, though not rigid, structure for therapy and upholding it, and by demonstrating that I value my own time and word. To illustrate the kinds of issues that can emerge I have constructed composite case examples of five types of client reactions to the requirement that they pay for missed sessions–angry, passive, compliant, responsible, and distressed–into which I have incorporated discussion of related countertransference issues.

In therapy, I work from the feminist principle of illuminating–not reinforcing–power differences, so the policing tone of the word "enforce" creates discomfort for me. At the same time, the term most accurately reflects my feeling about performing this difficult task. The tension resulting when power is both held and exposed is perhaps one of the most difficult aspects to manage in the therapeutic dynamic. Thus, policy is enforced by authority of the therapist's position and the vulnerability of the client in the therapy, while the therapist knows and the client may understand that the client is able to disempower the therapist by withdrawing from therapy.

PSYCHOLOGICAL APPROACH TO UNDERSTANDING

In developing my understanding of the complexities of this issue, I have drawn from various approaches to psychoanalytic thought, relying on the work of Robert Stolorow and his colleagues (Stolorow,

Brandchaft & Atwood, 1987) for some basic principles. Their reformulation of fundamental psychoanalytic principles is compatible with my own thinking and my feminist perspective, although theirs is not a feminist analysis. The fundamental position of these theorists differs from other psychoanalytic approaches in that it emphasizes the intersubjective field created when two "subjectivities" intersect. They believe neither that a therapist is able to achieve and maintain a position of neutrality nor that particular concepts are true in all cases (and thus "concretized"). Their position has implications for basic psychoanalytic principles including transference and countertransference. The authors caution against concretizing the notion of transference as regression to a reenactment of an earlier experience, displacement to the therapist of emotions that have been repressed, projection, or distortion of reality. Rather, they understand transference as "a microcosm of the patient's total psychological life . . . an expression of the *continuing influence* of organizing principles and imagery that crystallized out of the patient's early formative experiences" (Stolorow et al., 1987, p. 36). According to these authors, it is essential that the client's subjective perspective is always the starting point for understanding. From this perspective, "the analysis of transference provides a focal point around which the patterns dominating his [*sic*] existence as a whole can be clarified, understood, and thereby transformed" (p. 36). Countertransference is understood not as something generated by the client's pathology but a manifestation of the therapist's organizing principles and psychological structures. Countertransference and transference are viewed as "an intersubjective system of reciprocal mutual influence" (p. 42) which means the organizing principles of the therapist and client interact and influence each other, forming a unique intersubjective field.

My thinking has also been guided by behavioral principles, drawing from the work of Wachtel (1997) who integrated psychoanalytic and behavioral principles. Wachtel believes that behaviorism provides the means to "actively intervene in the human dilemmas that psychoanalysis has enabled us to understand . . . " (p. 5). In my discussion of case examples the power of modeled behavior is fully in evidence and gives pause to reflect on the importance of therapists continuing to develop their self-knowledge.

POLICY AS PROMISE

A promise is assurance given from one person to another that the other has a right to expect a particular action will take place. This is the underlying assumption of a scheduled appointment for therapy, that the therapist will reserve the period of time agreed upon exclusively for the client and will schedule no other appointments for that time. In accepting the promise, the client agrees to attend during the designated time so the two can consult for her or his benefit. The therapist is entrusted to keep the promise but has the additional responsibility to protect the promise from unconscious challenges made by the client, which sometimes come in the form of canceled or forgotten appointments. These unconscious challenges are usually signals that the client is experiencing a difficulty which she or he is unable to articulate. It is the responsibility of the client, in accepting the promise, to give appropriate notice, to turn up for the appointment, or to pay the fee. The failure of the woman in the opening paragraph to mention her obligation to pay shifted the responsibility back to me to remind her. Part of my work in keeping my promise was to help this client honor her acceptance of the promise, which she was unable to do at the time, for reasons we did not yet understand.

Promises are often problematic for clients who may have experienced countless unkept promises as children and adults. Past experiences of broken promises may have led the client to undervalue the promise of a scheduled appointment and to expect it to be undervalued. As the therapy progresses, an increasing and possibly conflicted dependency on the therapist and her promise to be present at the sessions may develop. Therefore, it is important in making policy that the practitioner determines exactly what the agreement will be, taking into consideration her own needs along with those of the client. However compassionate it may seem to allow client self-determination in matters of keeping appointments, or, on the other hand, how punitive it may seem to set and enforce a policy, caring for clients includes providing them with a clear statement of the promise made to them along with the implications of their acceptance of it. Conceptualizing appointment-setting and policy as a promise removes them from the realm of punitive interactions and places them in the realm of assisting the therapy process.

COUNTERTRANSFERENCE AND THE ANGRY CLIENT

Therapists think of themselves as helpers, not enforcers, so strong feelings can arise when it becomes necessary to stand firm on policy requiring payment for missed sessions. The nature of those feelings and the ways they are understood and managed can profoundly affect the course of therapy. One of the most difficult hurdles can occur if the therapist anticipates a client's anger. If she struggles with anger-related issues in her own life, the anticipation of a client's anger may bring her fears to the surface and possibly interfere with her ability to stand firm on policy. A client I shall call "Darleen" touched off such a dilemma.

Darleen was a woman in her mid-30s who spent her life, outside her workplace, in near-isolation because she was afraid of her own anger. In her sessions, we had discovered that her anger had developed much earlier in life as protection after she was sexually abused and its force had intensified as she became increasingly aware of the sexism that existed in her work world. However, it had come to dominate her emotional life and feel unmanageable. Clinicians have often observed that victim/survivors internalize or identify with their aggressors and begin to act towards others in highly aggressive ways (Davies & Frawley, 1994; McCann & Pearlman, 1990), something Darleen had done throughout her life in reality and imagination. The two intimate relationships in her past ended when she came close to violence, though she had always stopped herself before actually becoming physically violent. In apparent contradiction to her aggressive outbursts, Darleen was unable to say "no" to requests made of her which resulted in her adoption of an attitude of resentment towards most people in her life and a feeling of being victimized.

Darleen had canceled her appointment the morning of her session because she had scheduled a dental appointment at the same time. When she arrived at my office the following week she did not mention the incident. Her omission left the choice and responsibility with me to remind her or to make an exception. Considering Darleen's emotional history, my anticipation of an angry response to the news that I would be holding to my policy was not surprising. More unexpected and worrisome was my own feeling about confronting her with this news. As the moment drew near, I felt the rush of energy that signals fear and knew that my countertransference was active, dredging up the angry and unpredictable figures from my past that could still unnerve me at times. I wondered if Darleen would glare at me, become angry, or walk out. I was being confronted by my own feelings but also recognized that my concerns were rooted in the reality of this client's potential for violence. Aside from apprehension about Darleen's anger I worried that a confrontation could truncate her therapy. I vacillated between roles: I was simultaneously the enforcer, the victim, protector, and therapist. The challenge I faced–to manage my feelings while carrying out the intervention I believed to be in her best interests–was hardly unique, but I felt like a pioneer in uncharted territory. Intuitively, I sensed it was important to be firm with my policy, to bring structure to the intersubjective field, rather than manage the issue in a more collaborative manner, as I might do under other circumstances.

In those moments I also understood the importance of this event to my development as a therapist. The gnawing archaic question of the value of my services floated into consciousness and hovered. I entertained the possibility of suggesting a reduced rate for the missed session, questioned the wisdom of my decision to enforce my policy, and probed my memory for supervisors' teachings, or for readings or discussions that would either endorse my position or support an amendment to my policy, this one time. Knowing that Darleen longed to feel loved I considered the possible benefit of enacting the role of nurturing parent by waiving my fee, an option that reflects the struggle of many women therapists who feel obliged to take on the role of nurturer, sometimes at great personal sacrifice. Such selflessness is consistent with personal relationships in which women's caring is expected, no matter what the cost to them (Bograd, 1991; Philipson, 1993). The expectation is that because women are "naturally caring" they should provide services without payment or they should accept less payment than would a man in similar circumstances. My profession makes a worthwhile recommendation that members provide a portion of their services pro bono, but it is important to be clear, in each case, about the reasons for doing so, otherwise women risk colluding in their own subordination, and the implicit message to other women will be that they should do the same.

Ultimately, I recognized my fears and attempts to divert from the path I needed to take, and agreed with Furlong (1992) from whose work I inferred that failing to charge for this session would have constituted acting out my wish to avoid Darleen's anger. Still, I was tempted to flee from this responsibility and felt concerned about my capacity to hold her anger and remain fully present for her. I knew that I needed to ride the waves of her anger without fleeing emotionally, without compromising my integrity or becoming resentful. If I failed to act on my cancellation policy I might have sustained an unconscious resentment of my client and disappointment in myself, an unhealthy mixture the best antidote for which is to act from an ethic of self-care. In this instance, self-care meant staying with the policy I had established for occasions such as this.

Imagining myself in Darleen's position, I knew that she, too, needed this opportunity. For her, the challenge would be to work through her anger safely and non-aggressively with the very person whom, in that moment, she would view as another soft-voiced oppressor asking for her compliance. In this, I am not implying that provoking anger in a client is justifiable. Rather, I knew intuitively that Darleen would be angry and that she often felt anger she did not express and could not resolve, leaving it to fester and foment inside. If I had taken another approach such as exploring with her at length the issue of payment, we may have been spared the expression of her anger in the session and she may have taken responsibility for payment. It seemed likely, however, that she would have felt shamed or manipulated and resentful, a conclusion I reached thinking about her frequent references to the lengthy, seductive conversations used by the woman who had sexually abused her to manipulate her into complying. Moreover, if I had let my fears prevent me from standing firm on my policy, I would have inadvertently reinforced her sense of being the aggressor, a part of herself that she feared and disliked, and she would have been left with a model of fear rather than strength. Keeping these things in mind, I decided to enforce my policy, carefully and straightforwardly, treating her simply as an adult involved in a transaction with another adult. I both feared and hoped that in response she would express her anger, and hoped that I would be strong enough to contain it while helping her to explore all its components both present and past. If, instead, I became preoccupied with concerns about myself in this session, I would be unable to tend to her needs or to maintain "sustained empathic inquiry" (Stolorow et al., 1987) in order to explore the meaning of this event for her.

When I reminded Darleen of the policy she became angry and emphasized that she needed the dental work and had been able to take advantage of a cancellation rather than waiting months for an appointment. I explained that I supported her care of her health as well as her freedom to make choices, but in assuming I would overlook my fee for the missed session she was asking me to bear responsibility for her decision. Darleen's expression softened and her mood shifted as she began to understand the reasons for my position, and we were able to begin the emotional process of exploring the meaning of these events. During the months that followed I noticed that Darleen was interacting with increasing self-assurance, vacillating less between the aggressor and victim positions. In one session she volunteered the information that she was modeling her behavior after the assertiveness I demonstrated in the enforcement session.

While the acquisition of insight is important in therapy it became evident in my work with Darleen that behavior modeled by the therapist is also an integral part of the work. Darleen could see, hear, and feel the impact of someone doing what she had not been able to do. My modeling was meaningful to Darleen because it occurred in the context of an intersubjective field in which I was functioning under conditions analogous to those of difficult periods of her life. She was not simply watching me perform; she could relate to me and what I was doing at a deep emotional level. She believed she could hurt me. She knew that I knew of her aggression but faced her, nonetheless, and survived. She saw my vulnerability and my strength. At the same time, she was the recipient of my assertive behavior and found the interaction to be safe for her. Applying these observations meant she could act the same way–she could state outright in a reasonable way what her position was, or ask for what she needed–without fearing that she might hurt, or be hurt, by the other person. She was able to participate in and observe the interaction from the recipient and the agent positions.

Orange, Atwood, and Stolorow (1997) distinguish between two manifestations of the repetitive dimension of the transference. In one, the client longs to have something supplied that has been missing; in the other, the client seeks an antidote for something "crushingly present." Darleen may have wished for me to provide a form of caring by relieving her of responsibility for the missed session. If I had done so she may have internalized the notion that her aggression could terrify me as it terrified her. As Raney (1986) suggested, fee arrangements can mean, symbolically, that the therapist is able to withstand or contain the client's aggression. By maintaining my position in the face of Darleen's aggression I modeled a calm fearlessness and demonstrated to both of us that her aggression was not so powerful; sitting alone with her in my office I could face it and survive. I did not allow it to terrorize me as it had terrorized her for so many years. By modeling assertiveness in the face of her anger I provided her with an alternative to the extremes of victim and aggressor between which she vacillated. In this behavioral way I addressed one repetitive dimension of her transference, the crushing presence of her aggression.

Although it seemed easier to overlook Darleen's obligation in the face of her anger, I knew that if I neglected to enforce my policy I might have felt victimized. As the victim of my own fear I might have experienced a certain amount of anger, resentment, and a vague sense of having been abused. For Darleen the interaction would have mimicked many other situations in her life in which she, the victim, had become the victimizer, a phenomenon that McCann and Pearlman (1990) refer to as a "disturbed power schema." Thus, canceling her appointment without sufficient notice, then failing to take responsibility for her actions, created exactly the right set of circumstances through which to access some of the deep issues that plagued her. She presented us with a situation through which to see the patterns that had snagged her and kept her bound up in a life of increasing despair, isolation, and hopelessness. These circumstances also presented me with a problem to work through in order to be effective with her.

HONORING PROCESS
TO MITIGATE COUNTERTRANSFERENCE

Even though feelings may be less intense than those just described, the countertransference can still be informative and the emergent issues highly significant. In the examples that follow, feelings of doubt, compassion and possibly over-identification with the client emerged when the issue of payment for a missed session was raised.

Barry was in his late 50s, and financially successful through a combination of business acumen and frugality. In the third month of his therapy, he called one afternoon to cancel his appointment for the following morning. When he arrived the following week he apologized for missing the appointment but made no reference to payment. My policy required that notification be given by noon of the day preceding the appointment, thus establishing a clear cut-off for cancellation calls. Since I had picked up messages at noon I knew he telephoned after the deadline but felt reluctant to address the issue of payment. Barry had only recently felt safe enough to begin working on difficult childhood issues and I felt it was important to continue uninterrupted. At the same time, I believed that the most valuable learning in therapy often took place by paying close attention to the process of sessions and exploring ruptures when they occurred. Thus, tentatively, I took up the subject of the late cancellation. To my surprise, Barry insisted he had made the cancellation within the appropriate time frame and was so firm about it that I began to doubt my perception of events. As the discussion continued it became evident that Barry's insistence was disproportionate to the event and I silently reaffirmed that I was correct in my understanding of the time frame. Shifting focus slightly, I began to inquire about the importance of money to Barry, something that had always been evident but which we had never addressed directly. He then disclosed that his stepfather, who had lived with the family from the time Barry was five, had exploited him. Throughout his school years, Barry was forced to work at menial and back-breaking tasks, then turn over his entire earnings to his stepfather. He also knew that his sister had been sexually abused by the man. His mother was in poor health, unable to work, and completely dependent on the stepfather for her own financial support as well as that of her four children. She could not leave him and so she and her children, including Barry, were captives of the man. Through the intersecting subjectivities of his childhood Barry learned to approach life and relationships with the expectation that he would be exploited and unprotected. He grew up determined never to allow himself to be financially dependent on another person but had taken this resolve to the extreme and would go to great lengths to avoid spending money, even to mis-remembering the time of a telephone call.

In a different case, a client named Ruth who had recently begun what would most surely become long-term therapy, did not show up for her weekly appointment. Her absence occurred the week after I canceled our appointment because of illness. When Ruth arrived for the next session she expressed incredulity at her forgetfulness; failing to keep a commitment was completely out of character for her. In her expression of amazement she did not, however, mention her obligation to pay for the missed session, therefore effectively shifting responsibility to me to raise the topic. I felt some reluctance to charge for the session because Ruth was so thoroughly distressed about missing it and had been an extremely conscientious client until that point. None the less, I resisted the urge to retreat into the nurturer role described in Darleen's case, and kept to my policy. Ruth responded with a plea, saying she had not intended to miss; in fact, she so looked forward to the appointments that she certainly would not miss one purposely. Although she did not state it outright, her implicit plea was: How can I be held responsible for payment, when I simply did not remember? I felt myself weaken, but gently reiterated the policy and elaborated on the rationale for it. A long pause followed, after which Ruth agreed to pay for the session. She then began to cry, protesting that she was being punished for forgetting. Carefully, I began to explore what Ruth was experiencing in the moment, and together we reviewed the events beginning with my illness. It emerged that Ruth had felt deeply distressed by my illness, even harboring a fear that her need, which felt enormous to her, had somehow caused it. To compensate for her inability to be a self-advocate asking directly for what she needed and wanted, she had developed a dependency on others, relying on them to anticipate her needs and fill the void she felt so deeply. Resorting to ways and means common to many women who have met with disenfranchisement, systemic disempowerment, or abuse, she learned to employ non-verbal and indirect methods to meet her needs. For example, in her sessions she attempted to satisfy her need for more of my attention by talking on at length after I announced the end of the session. This method of interacting made Ruth highly vulnerable since her needs were never adequately addressed or satisfied and relationships became strained. Thus her sense of emptiness increased, relationships felt unsafe, and she sustained feelings of guilt.

Ruth's situation was further complicated by her real fear of dependence. In her marriage, her husband had become her lifeline, and as a result she had come to resent and ultimately disrespect him because she needed him so much. She also believed he thought of her as a burden. She was conflicted, sometimes wanting to be like a little girl, fully dependent, while at other times wanting independence, but she did not know how to strike a balance between these needs and would often resort to devious and indirect methods in her attempts to get what she wanted. Since she did not approve of this behavior which she labeled "manipulative," she learned to supply a rational explanation for her behavior to save herself from her own critical judgment. Thus, she believed that if she could not understand her tears they must mean she was manipulating for attention. She had thoroughly internalized the cultural tendency to label women's emotions manipulative, making it hard for her to ask for support when she was feeling needy. Fearing that she had demanded too much of me, Ruth unconsciously attempted to ease the burden by forgetting one of her sessions and ease her guilt by depriving herself of the longed-for contact. The missed session was an expression of her deep distress and guilt that seemed rooted in a child-like sense of omnipotence. At the same time she wanted me to know about her distress, so I could comfort her and supply something that Ruth felt was missing (Orange et al., 1997). This wish manifested in her protest at being expected to pay for the session, with its implicit hope that I would understand her pain. As a rational adult she could not protest my illness, but she could protest being charged for something that was not her fault. The forgotten appointment had provided the vehicle for expression of the pain she felt in her need and dependency which was revealed when I protected the promise of the appointment from this unconscious challenge.

As Ruth and I sorted through the maze of her feelings during the following weeks she frequently expressed admiration for the way I had handled the payment issue saying that I had acted in a compassionate but firm way. Ruth was reassured by my failure to yield to her pleas, and commented that I had demonstrated assertive, limit-setting behavior such as she herself had never been able to achieve. She expressed sadness about her inability to be assertive, noting the emotional drain and ultimate resentment she experienced when she was unable to express her deepest feelings or ask directly for what she needed. She attributed her deficit in part to a lack of effective role models, a lament I had heard expressed many times by women struggling to change their personal situations and ways of interacting or to get ahead professionally.

THE PARADOX OF THE RESPONSIBLE CLIENT

When a client cancels late–that is, outside of the requested time frame–and voluntarily accepts responsibility to pay for the missed session the matter can be finished quickly. It would be erroneous, however, to assume the matter is resolved. On the contrary, a discussion about the client's choice to cancel the therapy session rather than make alternate arrangements might prove very fruitful in determining the value that the client places on the therapy. Quite likely the client places a high value on the therapy, but in some cases ready payment for a missed session means something different.

Greg, an entertainer, canceled a half hour before his appointment, then handed me cash for the missed session as well as the current one when he walked in the door the following week. As I accepted his payment I felt relieved–too relieved, I quickly realized. That instant flash of knowing, so easy to overlook, was something I had learned to trust so I heeded its signal to think about the implication of Greg failing to pay for the missed session and realized that the idea of a confrontation with this well-known client set off a feeling of apprehension. I understood that his quick payment and my relief suggested that a larger issue was being avoided so I began to probe Greg's feelings about paying for the session. His response was that it was "no big deal," and it was easier to pay the fee than argue about it. The previous week a friend had called and he had decided to miss the session in favor of drinks and a visit so the responsibility for the session was his. Moreover, the fee meant little to him. As I probed further it became clear that although he had attended several sessions he felt their usefulness was very limited, that the sessions–like the fee–meant little to him, and he was thinking about termination. He felt I was not challenging him enough and he would often leave sessions feeling he had simply entertained me while I had functioned as his audience, as did most other people in his life. As I continued to probe, encouraged by what I was hearing, Greg remarked that this session was different because I seemed more involved, and he felt hopeful we could work together after all.

AN EXCEPTION TO POLICY

Unlike the four cases just discussed, occasionally it is appropriate to make an exception to the policy as in the case I describe below. In general, this should not be done when a strong countertransference is present or without a full discussion of the reasons with the client. However, sometimes making an exception can assist the therapy process.

Rhoda was an on-call nurse in her mid-40s when she came to me for psychotherapy. Her past was dominated by an addiction to prescription drugs, which she claimed was a hazard of her profession. Her habit had been heavy and she had often broken the law using forgery and deceptive behavior to procure her supply. She had always managed to avoid detection but colleagues had become suspicious and Rhoda had lost their trust and friendship. When she realized that it was only a matter of time until she would be caught she admitted her problem, went into a detoxification unit and participated in brief, intense therapy. She successfully conquered her addiction problem but when she arrived at my office two years later, had reached a point where she felt emotionally stuck. We quickly developed a therapeutic rapport and embarked on a course of intense therapy. We set a regular appointment time at a day and hour that was least likely to conflict with any work she might be called to do. Usually she knew at least a day in advance if she had to work on the day of our appointment and she would call within the required time frame to cancel or reschedule her appointment. On the rare occasion that she could not cancel within the time frame she willingly paid for the missed appointment without being reminded. It happened, however, that she began to be called to work on shorter notice and was sometimes unable to give the required notice. In genuine distress she raised the issue as she paid for her third missed appointment in two months. She found the sessions valuable and she felt she was making progress, however, she was reluctant to pay for so many missed sessions and she could not afford to forfeit work in order to attend sessions. We discussed the issue at length and Rhoda proposed that she not be asked to pay if she had to miss a session because of a late call to work, but if she missed because she had forgotten to call on time she would pay. In response to her proposal I pointed out that she was asking me to trust her. Although she had not realized the implication of her request she thoughtfully agreed that she was, indeed, asking for my trust. In that context, I agreed to her proposal, and Rhoda never disappointed either of us.

Although Rhoda had managed to avoid being caught and criminalized, the issue of trust that she brought to therapy was not unlike that of women who have been through the criminal justice system and who have been labeled untrustworthy—whatever their crimes—by those of us who have learned not to trust (Sommers, 1995). She wanted and needed an opportunity to prove to herself and others that she could be trusted. The therapeutic context and the payment policy provided an opportunity for the mutual experience of trust-building that she needed in order to move ahead in her life.

DUAL VALUE: INSIGHT AND MODELING

The case examples illustrate the rich insights that can be gained when therapists explore the fertile ground of payment for missed sessions. Darleen realized the depth of her split between victim and oppressor roles which had forced her into near-isolation and profound despair. Barry discovered that in his attempts to avoid exploitation he had the capability of becoming an exploiter. Ruth got in touch with the depth of her need and her guilt about the ways she would try to have it satisfied. Greg uncovered his disdain for the very intersubjective reality that had contributed to his success. Rhoda discovered that her inability to continue developing emotionally was linked to a basic need for a trusting relationship. Thus, in these examples, when the difficult issue of payment was removed from the realm of dollars and cents and transformed through the lens of promise-keeping, global concepts such as aggression, fear, need, value, trust, commitment, and power emerged and the clinical value of addressing them could readily be understood.

In addition to exploring the ways in which confronting payment issues can lead to meaningful insights, the stories of Darleen, Barry, Ruth, Greg, and Rhoda illustrate the benefits that can accrue when therapists model assertive behavior. In the here-and-now of the therapy session clients can observe another individual placing value on her work, facing anger and devaluation of her work fearlessly, exploring to find truth in the presence of opposition, or resisting heart-wrenching manipulations. In the domain of fee for service these feats are especially meaningful because the therapist has something to lose that everyone can understand–her source of income.

It is equally important to consider the impact when therapists fail to enforce their policies. Since clients are keen observers of their therapists, the lack of enforcement–the failure to protect the promise–is as meaningful as the act of enforcing policy. The messages conveyed through the failure to act may include fear, indecisiveness, lack of self-care, and perhaps even unexpressed anger, all of which suggest that the therapist is unable to contain the difficult work of therapy and as such, threaten the very structure of therapy and derail the process.

Frequently, it is therapists' own unresolved and unintegrated organizing principles that obstruct their ability to conceptualize the issues in a global way, keeping them mired in the concrete world of money. Ironically, some of the most honorable-seeming organizing principles can contribute to these failures of therapy. For example, feelings of compassion and a wish to be altruistic when inappropriately acted upon, can direct a therapist away from the structure of policy and divert her onto a path that simply reinforces the very problems the client came to resolve. Whatever the organizing principle, or countertransference, that interferes with the work of therapy, whether it be a wish to nurture, a question of self worth, or unresolved fear, its essential function is to relieve the therapist of responsibility. When the therapist succumbs to the interference, rich opportunities to work at a deep and meaningful level can be missed. As the case examples illustrated, there are effective ways to stay on a therapeutic path including continuing development of one's awareness of countertransference issues, honoring therapeutic process, maintaining a healthy cynicism when difficult situations move ahead "too" smoothly, and making exceptions to process and policy only with extreme caution.

CONCLUSION

Beginning with a conceptualization of the scheduled appointment as a promise made between therapist and client, and payment policy as a way of protecting it, I have outlined some of the difficulties that arise when clients present unconscious challenges to payment policy. Using case examples, I have demonstrated sound clinical reasons for standing firm on payment for missed sessions when the requested notice of cancellation has not been given. In addition, I have described one case where it was therapeutically advantageous to make an exception to the policy. Countertransference issues arising when therapists were faced with enforcing policy were incorporated into the discussion. My hope in developing this discussion was to underscore the need for therapists to come to a clear understanding of their values and feelings about payment issues in therapy, to face the organizing principles that may stand in the way of their effectiveness with their clients in this important and fundamental aspect of therapy. For women therapists the additional struggle of a culture that pressures them to question their very right to earn a living from their work as helpers is an important obstacle to overcome.

Listening empathically to clients is the starting point in determining how payment issues, or any issues, are best managed. Since payment is an element of therapy that can level the intersubjective field because it strikes at the therapist's needs and vulnerabilities as well as those of the client, therapists must also listen carefully to themselves. My hope is that this discussion will encourage therapists to explore the many opportunities to add to meaningful experience in therapy presented by payment issues.

REFERENCES

Bograd, M. (1991). The Color of Money: Pink or Blue? In T. Goodrich (Ed.), *Women and Power: Perspectives for Family Therapy*. New York: W.W. Norton & Company.

Davies, J.M., & Frawley, M.G. (1994). *Treating the Adult Survivor of Childhood Sexual Abuse: A Psychoanalytic Perspective*. New York: Basic Books.

Furlong, A. (1992). Some Technical and Theoretical Considerations Regarding the Missed Session. *International Journal of Psycho-Analysis, 73*, 701-718.

Krueger, D. (Ed.). (1986). *The Last Taboo: Money as Symbol and Reality in Psychotherapy and Psychoanalysis*. New York: Brunner/Mazel.

McCann, I.L., & Pearlman, L.A. (1990). *Psychological Trauma and the Adult Survivor: Theory, Therapy, and Transformation*. New York: Brunner/Mazel.

Orange, D., Atwood, G., & Stolorow, R. (1997). *Working Intersubjectively: Contextualism in Psychoanalytic Practice*. Hillsdale, NJ: The Analytic Press.

Philipson, I. (1993). *On the Shoulders of Women: The Feminization of Psychotherapy*. New York: Guilford Press.

Raney, J. (1986). The Effect of Fees on the Course and Outcome of Psychotherapy and Psychoanalysis. In D. Krueger (Ed.), *The Last Taboo: Money as Symbol and Reality in Psychotherapy and Psychoanalysis*. New York: Brunner/Mazel.

Sommers, E. (1995). *Voices from Within: Women Who Have Broken the Law*. Toronto: University of Toronto Press.

Stolorow, R., Brandchaft, B., & Atwood, G. (1987). *Psychoanalytic Treatment: An Intersubjective Approach*. Hillsdale, NJ: The Analytic Press.

Wachtel, P. (1997). *Psychoanalysis, Behavior Therapy, and the Relational World*. Washington, DC: American Psychological Association.

Reflections
on the Symbolic and Real Meaning of Money
in the Relationship
Between the Female African American Client
and Her Therapist

Janet R. Brice-Baker

SUMMARY. This article focuses on the therapeutic relationship between female African American clients and female African American psychotherapists. The author is particularly interested in how issues related to self worth, a woman's definition of success, a woman's sense of her own power or powerlessness get acted out in this unique relationship. Historically, the idea of possessing money and the things that money can buy has been the domain and concern of men. Therefore, it is rather provocative to explore (1) the real and symbolic meaning of money for a group of people, namely African American women, who have been at the bottom of the economic hierarchy and (2) how those meanings impact the most intimate of relationships. This paper will attempt to look at this issue from both the client's and the therapist's points of view and suggest ways for therapists to handle some of these issues as they arise in therapy. *[Article copies available for a fee from The Haworth Document Delivery Service: 1-800-342-9678. E-mail address: getinfo@haworthpressinc.com <Website: http://www.haworthpressinc.com>]*

Janet R. Brice-Baker, PhD, is Assistant Professor in Clinical Psychology at the Yeshiva University Ferkauf Graduate School of Psychology. She is also a consultant to the New Jersey Department of Corrections, serving at the Edna Mahan Correctional Facility for Women.

Address correspondence to: Janet R. Brice-Baker, 81 Drake Road, Somerset, NJ 08873 (E-mail: dwbaker@castle.com).

[Haworth co-indexing entry note]: "Reflections on the Symbolic and Real Meaning of Money in the Relationship Between the Female African American Client and Her Therapist." Brice-Baker, Janet R. Co-published simultaneously in *Women & Therapy* (The Haworth Press, Inc.) Vol. 22, No. 3, 1999, pp. 69-80; and: *For Love or Money: The Fee in Feminist Therapy* (eds: Marcia Hill, and Ellyn Kaschak) The Haworth Press, Inc., 1999, pp. 69-80. Single or multiple copies of this article are available for a fee from The Haworth Document Delivery Service [1-800-342-9678, 9:00 a.m. - 5:00 p.m. (EST). E-mail address: getinfo@haworthpressinc.com].

KEYWORDS. African American, women, black, therapists, gender, socioeconomic status, psychotherapy

INTRODUCTION

Money has always been the subject of heated debate. However, the experience of having money and of not having money has had a different meaning to people depending on their gender, race, ethnicity and age. For many, the possession of a great deal of money by an individual is equated with success, power and privilege. When any two people are in a relationship, the person who has the money is most likely the person with the power in the relationship.

In the psychotherapeutic relationship, therapists have particularly wondered about what meaning to associate with a client's failure to pay for services, on time or at all. Therapists have also struggled with how to set fees, whether or not to offer their clients a sliding fee scale and when and how often is it appropriate to do pro bono work.

Research on therapy and counseling with African American clients has for some time focused predominantly on the issue of the importance of a racial match between the client and her therapist. Twenty years ago, a study by Sattler (as cited in Davis & Proctor, 1989) concluded that the choices made by African American clients were dictated more by the personal style of the therapist they worked with than the race of the therapist. Atkinson, Furlong, and Poston (as cited in Davis & Proctor, 1989) advanced this research even further with the addition of other variables. They found that African American clients did feel that having a therapist of the same race was important, but it was only important 55% of the time. Race ranked fifth in importance after therapist's level of education, similarity of attitude between therapist and client, older age and similarity in personality between therapist and client. Overall, the studies done throughout the years supported the idea that African American clients prefer an African American therapist when you control for non-racial therapist characteristics (Davis & Proctor, 1989).

The pool of African American clinical social workers, clinical psychologists and psychiatrists is very small. The number of African Americans who seek treatment far outnumber these professionals and therefore the likelihood of actually getting a racially matched dyad is small. The probability diminishes even more if one tries to match the

African American client and African American therapist on other variables as well. A match on socioeconomic status may not be a desire of the client. However, my informal discussions with female African American colleagues strongly points to the subject of economics, as it relates to power and individual worth, as having a powerful positive and negative impact on the therapeutic relationship.

This article will focus on the socioeconomic differences and similarities between the African American client and her African American female therapist. Hopefully, these clinical observations and hypotheses will raise the level of awareness of therapists about the meaning of money in this unique relationship.

SYMBOLISM: TRANSFERENCE AND COUNTERTRANSFERENCE

Transference has been defined as "the experiencing by the patient of affects, perceptions, attitudes and fantasies in the therapeutic interaction. These do not derive from the therapist but are a repetition of reactions originating in the patient's past and unconsciously displaced onto the therapist" (Kernberg, 1984, p. 266). Psychodynamic therapy has been noted for its attention to and interpretation of the relationship between therapist and client. Money can certainly be a part of the gestalt that a client forms about her therapist.

Countertransference, on the other hand, refers to "all emotional reactions the therapist has to the patient" (as cited in Kernberg, 1984, p. 69). "These countertransferential reactions can include reactions to the transference, reactions to the patient, reactions to events in the patient's life and reaction to events in the therapist's own life" (as cited in Kernberg, 1984, p. 69-70).

Historically, African Americans have been thought of and treated as a relatively homogenous group. Little attention has been given to variables which might, in other contexts, account for the variability among people. Socioeconomic differences within the African American community is one such variable. In part, the failure to admit that these types of differences exist and to examine them stems from stereotyped images of all African Americans as poor people; basically a people of the underclass. Perhaps we do not know enough about how these differences get played out in general or in the therapy room.

Consider the African American female therapist who may enter the therapy room with a number of conscious and unconscious issues related to money. If she is conscious of these issues they may begin to manifest themselves in the questions she asks herself: Should I be embarrassed by my income relative to that of my client when that client is Black? Am I only comfortable with African American clients who are in the same socioeconomic category as myself because the poorer ones make me feel guilty about what I have? If I do feel guilty about what I have achieved and what I have acquired, what do I do to assuage that guilt?

Clinical Vignette 1
(Names have been changed to protect confidentiality)

Dr. Martin was a 28 year old, single African American psychologist practicing in a large community mental health center on the poorer side of Boston. Seventy-five percent of her caseload was indigent; comprised of both Blacks and Whites. This was her second job. When Dr. Martin graduated and got her first job she made what she considered an "investment" in good work clothes. Her mother had always impressed upon her and her siblings the fact that there were clothes for school, for work, for church and for play. You were always supposed to keep them separate. Little by little she acquired her suits, dresses, shoes and handbags. She bought Evan Picone, Liz Claiborne and Jones of New York suits in the "better sportswear" department. Her shoes were from 9 West and Aigner. Her purse and briefcase were Coach. It goes without saying that she had matching hose and accessories. When Dr. Martin stepped into the office she felt like she was appropriately attired. She felt good about the way she looked. She continued to have that feeling when she saw her poor White clients, middle class White clients and middle class Black clients. However, whenever she began therapy with a new Black client, who also happened to be poor, she felt a tremendous sense of anxiety and guilt. Some of these clients seemed to make it a point to begin each session by commenting on her appearance.

What could have been going on with Dr. Martin? Some African American therapists, by virtue of their education, and by extension, their earning power, have been the ones to bring their families squarely into the ranks of the middle class. Some African American therapists are grappling with having come, not too long ago, from families just as poor as some of their clients. They may view their clothes as a sort of uniform, or more accurately, a coat of armor. The outfit gives them legitimacy. "If I look like a professional therapist then everyone will believe that I am one." When faced with a poor African American family/client, someone like Dr. Martin may feel a type of "survivor" guilt stemming from the fact that despite the most rampant racism in America she was still able to achieve and become successful.

Clinical Vignette 2

Another therapist spoke of her reluctance to wear her diamond engagement ring to work. She stated that on a number of occasions her poorer clients commented on the ring and asked questions about its size and cost. In some instances the African American women took the ring to be a symbol of the fact that you were loved and the extent to which you were loved by your spouse. For African American women who have been in abusive relationships and suffer from low self-esteem, such fantasized gestures on the part of African American men have powerful meaning for them.

This therapist and Dr. Martin both expressed the sentiment that certain statements from less affluent African American clients left them feeling guilty about what they had acquired. Some therapists respond in the following ways: they refrain from wearing expensive jewelry to work, they wear their jewelry but when comments are made about it they downplay its value ("this isn't real gold," etc.), they "dress down" when going to the office or try overly hard to form an alliance with the client on the basis of racial issues (a desire they would not have necessarily felt if the African American client had money).

Let's examine some of these responses and their possible consequences. Refraining from wearing real (vs. costume) jewelry or attempting to lessen its value seems like an effort on the part of the therapist to "level the playing field." If that is in fact the therapist's motivation, one has to question its success. Such action on the part of the therapist does not automatically imbue the client with more worth nor does it make the therapist and client equal in terms of power. The only thing it does is temporarily relieve the therapist of her feelings of guilt.

The therapist who tries to overcompensate for the difference in economic status between herself and her client by being overly sympathetic on racial issues can do the client a disservice. In this instance the therapist runs the risk of losing sight of intrapsychic/personality issues. The client who senses the therapist's discomfort with her socio-economic status and by extension her position may try to induce guilt in that therapist to avoid the exploration of issues not having to do with race. In other words, the client may use the therapist's overcompensating behaviors to divert the focus of therapy so it is solely about race.

Other overcompensating behaviors could include not discussing the client's failure to pay or automatically lowering the customary fee simply because the client is another African American and not because the therapist has assessed a legitimate financial need.

The remedy for many of these issues lies in individual supervision, group supervision or peer consultation of cases. But in order to be effective, the topics in supervision cannot be considered individually and consecutively. The supervisor cannot talk about how the therapist feels about the client's race on one day and then on a separate day discuss the therapist's feelings about the client's socioeconomic status. They have to be discussed in tandem. How do you feel about the African American client who is middle class, rich or poor? Why does working with poor African American clients elicit guilt that is not present when working with a poor White client? What does it mean for the therapist to take money for services she is providing to members of her own race? Is the African American therapist saying something about her own self-esteem if she charges her clients less than her White colleagues would?

THE CLIENT'S VIEW

A key question in therapy is what meaning should be given to or what issue should be explored when the African American client does not pay for therapy. Some African American clients believe that a therapist who is also African American should not charge a fee but donate her services to the African American community. This can stem from a belief in a world view that stresses working together for the good of all (Sue & Sue, 1981). A derivative of that collective thinking is the notion that African Americans who succeed have an obligation to give back to the people who have nurtured, supported them and made their success possible.

Others may refuse or neglect to pay for treatment as a way to devalue treatment; something also done by many clients who are not African Americans. The difference, however, may be in the reason behind devaluing the treatment. Historically, the theoretical underpinnings of psychotherapeutic intervention have neglected the needs and issues of people of color (Boyd-Franklin, 1989). In many situations, those same theories have been used to label and pathologize the behavior of African American clients.

In another situation, not paying for treatment can be seen as a way to devalue the African American therapist who may be seen as having been corrupted by her education and training in predominantly White institutions of learning. Tangible signs of relative wealth on the part of the therapist (type of clothing worn, jewelry, how hair is done, whether or not nails are professionally manicured, type of car driven, etc.) may be seen as symbols of that corruption.

Failure to pay can also be conceptualized in terms of outright rejection of the therapist but not necessarily the therapeutic process. An African American client may view an African American therapist as less qualified than a White therapist. This way of thinking has been conceptualized as a form of internalized racism (Greene, 1993).

The transferential valence can be positive as well as negative. Many African American female clients need and seek positive role models. The therapist is one of the people in their lives who may provide modeling. Many see the therapist's education as a sign that African American women can and have made it in a White, male dominated world. Manifestations of the therapist's income can be taken as a sign of that woman's ability, and the ability of her race and gender, to be successful.

There are other things which may come together to influence the symbolism behind money. It is worthwhile to consider to what extent a client believes that having money serves as a protective force against racism. Some clients have had the experience that money, no matter how it has been obtained, is equated with power. Power is seen as influence and the only safeguard against becoming a victim of racism. For other clients, the link is less direct between having money and freedom from racism. Money can be seen as a direct consequence of education and it is therefore the knowledge that serves as protection. How does one translate the meaning of "protection"? Does having money remove one from being the target of racism or does having money enable you to strike back once you have been the target? This has been illustrated by some of my clients who have said, "I guess being a doctor and all you don't have to put up with none of this racial stuff." Others have expressed the sentiment in this way, "I suppose if any of these White folks bother you, you can afford to get yourself good legal representation and get justice."

A frequent issue that comes up in the psychotherapy of women is the quality of their self-esteem. To what extent is low self-esteem manifested in some African American women by their failure to pay for treatment they can well afford? And what about the African American women who never become clients because they see treatment as too much of a luxury? In other cases, they do not seek treatment when they can afford it because it could be viewed as an act of selfishness.

To a large extent, the negative stereotypes promulgated about African American men, women, children and the families they have formed have put African American women on the defensive. They are afraid of being accused of usurping the man's role in the family. Many of my clients have expressed concern that their financial success has been at the cost of the African American male's success. In some of these situations, therapy sessions have been devoted to discussing ways in which the woman has tried to play down or sabotage that success, particularly when in the presence of men.

The historical pattern of the African American female's subordination to the White male can encourage some African American clients to have doubts about how they and their therapists have established financial security. Some women have questioned whether or not they have really achieved anything on their own. Major concerns are expressed about the extent to which one has "prostituted" (both literally and figuratively) themselves to the White male.

Clearly, the issues mentioned above do not represent or characterize all relationships between African American female therapists and their African American female clients. Nonetheless, this is a particularly important discussion because historically, women, regardless of race, and African Americans, regardless of gender, have not enjoyed as equal an access to money as other groups. The female gender has traditionally been expected to have little to do with the handling of money. And African Americans have not yet achieved economic parity with their White counterparts. Add to the equation the fact that the particular profession of psychotherapy does not include training its practitioners to view what they do as a business.

MODERATING VARIABLES

There are certain variables that can moderate the extent to which the transferential and countertransferential issues around money and race will effect the therapeutic relationship. One such variable is racial identity. Several theoreticians and researchers have proffered a model of racial identity development (Cross, 1995; Helms, 1995). For the purposes of this paper, I will refer to the Cross model. Pre-encounter is considered the first stage of his 5-stage model. In this stage, an African American individual accepts and internalizes values of the dominant Eurocentric culture. A client in this stage of development is likely to devalue the African American therapist and value the White therapist. An extension of that devaluation can be manifested in a refusal to pay for services or being slow to pay. The second stage is "encounter" and during this stage the African American (or other minority) individual begins to experience cognitive dissonance. Usually this dissonance is an outgrowth of having experiences with members of her own race that contradict the negative stereotypes she has internalized. Money issues for a client at this stage emerge when she begins to see the African American therapist as someone worthy of being paid for her services. This could come from gaining knowledge of the therapist's credentials or it could come from staying in therapy long enough to judge, first hand, the quality of the therapist's work.

Immersion/emersion is a stage in Cross' model characterized by the minority individual's desire to surround herself with all that pertains to her race/ethnicity. At this stage there is overwhelming acceptance of all things African American and a rejection of all things White or Eurocentrically influenced. An African American client at this stage is likely to have a very positive transference to her African American therapist and look upon the therapist's possessions and other indications of financial success as a good thing.

In the fourth and fifth stages, internalization and commitment respectively, the minority individual has a solid core of racial identity which allows her to make decisions about people based on who they are and what they do rather than on their skin color alone. The therapist who needs her designer clothes, jewelry and luxury car to feel

"O.K." about herself has not reached this stage of development. The same can be said for the therapist who feels that she has to apologize to her Black clients for what she has accomplished and earned.

But the racial identities of the client and therapist are not the only moderating variables. A therapist cannot make interpretations about the meaning of money to a client in a vacuum. Other moderating variables include: the socioeconomic status of the client, the ease or difficulty the client has paying for therapy, the personality traits of the client, the number of generations a client's family has experienced some degree of financial security/success, and the client's viewpoint about whether psychotherapy is something worth paying for.

SUGGESTIONS FOR THERAPISTS

The symbolic and real meaning of money in the relationship between a client and her therapist is not an insurmountable obstacle. The following is a list of suggestions to begin addressing the concrete money issues as well as the symbolic:

1. Be very clear about your policies for payment. This is not to suggest that the therapist has to be rigid. Clarity and flexibility are two separate issues. African American female clients should be treated like any other client to the extent that the therapist is forthright about how fees are set (whether or not the therapist has a sliding scale), acceptable forms of payment (cash, personal checks, credit cards) and whether or not you will delay full payment, take a co-payment and wait for reimbursement from an insurance company. What can be offensive to all African American women is having the therapist assume that they cannot pay the regular fee solely on the basis of the fact that they are African American, rather than taking into consideration their circumstances.
2. Be sure to explain the consequences for late payment, failure to pay and missed sessions. These three situations should be addressed as soon as possible. Like any other client, consideration can be given to any change in financial circumstances that might affect the timeliness of payment or the ability to pay at all. This can be part of a discussion with the client. One of the things the therapist should be alert for is the presence or absence of discre-

tionary funds. If discretionary funds are available, how are they being utilized? Historically, we have been bombarded with negative and stereotyped images of African American people, as a whole, and poor African Americans, in particular, as wasteful or foolhardy with money. Once it has been established that the money is there, the therapist needs to elicit from the client how she is making decisions about the allocation of discretionary money. In some cases, African American women are using that money to help other people and in some cases they are using it for themselves. This line of inquiry usually pulls for themes about nurturance or the lack of nurturance in the client's life. Rather than condemning the present expenditure as frivolous (which is judgmental), the therapist has the opportunity to stress the idea of psychotherapy as something the woman can do for herself, a form of self care. African American women have been socialized to be caretakers of their own race as well as caretakers of members of the dominant White race (Greene, 1994). So, having the African American woman examine the extent to which she will take care of herself becomes more than just a gender issue, but a racial one as well.

3. Give the client an opportunity to tell you what obstacles, if any, she has in meeting her financial obligations.

4. Try not to ignore comments about your status and the things that you have. Even if these statements are made at the very beginning or end of a session it is not simply "polite conversation."

5. Therapists must be able to deal with the reality that, depending on the type of practice you do have, some of your African American clients will be significantly less well off than you while others may be in a better situation.

6. Therapists should be prepared to deal with the rejection and or anger of some clients around their socioeconomic differences.

7. Explore clients' fantasies about what they think money enables a person to do.

8. Therapists need to be prepared to respond to clients who believe that professionals should give back to the community by not charging fees. Initially, the client's definition of "giving back" needs to be clarified. Next, the therapist needs to find out why having a fee for service is viewed in this context. A possible response to a client could be, "It's interesting that you see it that

way. Others might characterize an African American's employment in a predominantly White-run institution as a form of giving to African Americans who would otherwise see White therapists." Another response might be, "I wonder if you could elaborate on this and envision the survival of the African American community if professionals in their ranks never charged for their services." A blanket belief on the part of African American women that African American professionals should provide free services and only pay Whites and/or men is a form of internalized sexism and racism. Such a statement says something about the perception of the relative worth of services coming from Whites vs. African Americans and men vs. women.

REFERENCES

Boyd-Franklin, N. (1989). *Black families in therapy.* New York: Guilford Press.

Cross, W. E. (1995). The psychology of Nigrescence: Revising the Cross model. In J. G. Ponterotto, J.M. Casas, L.A. Suzuki & C.M. Alexander (Eds.), *Handbook of multicultural counseling* (pp. 93-122). Thousand Oaks, California: Sage.

Davis, L.E., & Proctor, E.K. (1989). *Race, gender and class: Guidelines for practice with individuals, families and groups.* Englewood Cliffs, New Jersey: Prentice Hall.

Greene, B.A. (1993). Psychotherapy with African American women: Integrating feminist and psychodynamic models. *Journal of Training and Practice in Professional Psychology, 7*(1), 49-66.

Helms, J.E. (1995). An update of Helm's White and people of color racial identity models. In J. G. Ponterotto, J.M. Casas, L.A. Suzuki & C.M. Alexander (Eds.) *Handbook of multicultural counseling* (pp. 181-198). Thousand Oaks, California: Sage.

Kernberg, L. (1984). *Severe personality disorders: Psychotherapeutic strategies.* New Haven: Yale University Press.

Sue, D.W., & Sue, D. (1981). *Counseling the culturally different.* New York: John Wiley and Sons.

Barter:
Ethical Considerations
in Psychotherapy

Marcia Hill

SUMMARY. The use of barter as a method of payment in psychotherapy carries a number of risks, including that of exploiting the client and complicating and possibly damaging the therapeutic relationship. However, barter is one way of increasing the availability of therapy, respecting class differences, and avoiding the problems associated with using insurance for payment. The author proposes factors to consider in order to barter ethically in therapy: (1) the nature of the transference, (2) the kind of dual relationship created, (3) the economic context, (4) the relative cost of the barter to each participant, (5) other therapist-client power differences, and (6) the problem of evaluation. *[Article copies available for a fee from The Haworth Document Delivery Service: 1-800-342-9678. E-mail address: getinfo@haworthpressinc.com <Website: http://www.haworthpressinc.com>]*

KEYWORDS. Barter, psychotherapy, ethics

Although barter predates the invention of money by millennia, in late twentieth century Western civilization barter has come to be so unusual as to seem subversive. In cultures in which currency is the

Marcia Hill, EdD, is a psychologist in private practice in a rural area and co-editor of *Women & Therapy.*

Address correspondence to: Marcia Hill, 25 Court Street, Montpelier, VT 05602.

[Haworth co-indexing entry note]: "Barter: Ethical Considerations in Psychotherapy." Hill, Marcia. Co-published simultaneously in *Women & Therapy* (The Haworth Press, Inc.) Vol. 22, No. 3, 1999, pp. 81-91; and: *For Love or Money: The Fee in Feminist Therapy* (eds: Marcia Hill, and Ellyn Kaschak) The Haworth Press, Inc., 1999, pp. 81-91. Single or multiple copies of this article are available for a fee from The Haworth Document Delivery Service [1-800-342-9678, 9:00 a.m. - 5:00 p.m. (EST). E-mail address: getinfo@haworthpressinc.com].

only accepted standard of exchange, barter challenges capitalism by the simple expedient of not participating. Barter eliminates the impersonal character of most purchases. It does away with most or all of the systems that come between people in an exchange, systems that skim off a portion of the value of goods or services by offering packaging or access or advertising. Because it is a direct exchange between people, barter reminds us of what we are doing: exchanging the results of our time and skill for that of another person.

As methods of payment for psychotherapy have become increasingly Byzantine, many therapists have looked for alternatives to the difficulties of using insurance. While limited in scope, barter is one such alternative, one that avoids pre-authorization, billing, extension of benefit requests, worries about confidentiality, and even diagnoses. We would do well to consider it as one option in a range of payment possibilities.

PROS AND CONS OF USING BARTER

In addition to the benefits of offering an alternative economic system and avoiding the use of insurance to pay for therapy, barter's primary value in therapy is that it increases access to therapy in a respectful way. The Feminist Therapy Institute's ethical guidelines state clearly that "a feminist therapist increases her accessibility to and for a wide range of clients from her own and other identified groups through flexible delivery of services" (1987). The expense of therapy is a significant barrier to the availability of therapy for a number of people, particularly for those who are uninsured, underinsured, or unwilling to use insurance benefits which may compromise their privacy. Even a copayment or deductible may be beyond the financial reach of many.

Many therapists solve the dilemma of economic barriers to accessibility by offering services for free, for a reduced fee, or by forgiving all or part of the deductible or copayment. This can be a good solution, but it also carries risks. The client may feel infantilized, ashamed, or that she is obligated to the therapist, i.e., that she or he should not make too many emotional demands, should be grateful, should not be angry, and so forth (Drellich, 1991; Shainess, 1991). In addition, those clients who have been taken advantage of by caretakers may feel appropriately confused and insecure about boundaries; to see such a client for free can add to her or his anxiety and confusion. The therapist who accepts a low or no fee may feel resentful, particularly in response to what she or he perceives as any additional need on the part of the client, and may feel inclined to suggest less time-consuming or emotionally demanding forms of therapy regardless of their appropriateness. Parvin and Anderson (1995) note that "the client's ability to pay for therapy, rather than the client's needs, may drive decisions about whether a person will get therapy . . . and what method of therapy will be used" (p. 57). A therapist who feels fairly paid is more likely to be a generous and thoughtful caretaker, and models financial self-care for the client. A client who feels that she or he is paying fairly for services is potentially more able to ask for what she or he needs from the therapist, and may feel a greater sense of power and control in the therapy, as well as a healthy pride in paying her or his own way. Barter has the potential of avoiding these difficulties with reducing or forgiving the fee, and can allow the therapist to feel fairly compensated and the client to feel honorable about paying her or his way.

Socioeconomic class is central to the question of bartering. Individuals more likely to use barter–those with limited incomes, in rural areas, or who value barter as a lifestyle alternative (Parvin & Anderson, 1995)–are often those less likely to have the luxury of obtaining what they need or want with money. As I have argued elsewhere (Hill, 1995):

> To insist on being paid with money is to ignore the reality of how difficult it may be for some people to come by money. It is classist to assume (without other evidence) that difficulty in paying the fee, even a reduced fee, is necessarily some form of therapeutic resistance. (p. 78)

The Feminist Therapy Institute Code of Ethics (1987) states that "a feminist therapist is aware of the meaning and impact of her own ethnic and cultural background, gender, *class* [italics added], and sexual orientation." Awareness of the impact of class implies a responsiveness to the reality of limited economic resources; respect regarding class differences calls for an openness to alternative forms of payment.

However, despite the foregoing arguments in support of barter, the difficulties inherent in bartering in the context of therapy are substantial. Parvin and Anderson (1995) summarize these concerns as "the complexity of the relationship issues it [i.e., barter] raised and the potential for exploitation to occur" (p. 61). A review of the literature for barter in psychotherapy revealed exactly one article (Hendricks), written in 1979, describing bartering practices which were reflective of the Zeitgeist but some of which would universally be considered unethical today, such as bartering for personal services. Apparently, therapists have largely responded to the complexities of bartering with avoidance and silence.

The primary concern about bartering in psychotherapy is the danger of exploiting the client, and that danger is considerable. In bartering agreements outside of therapy, any concerns about exploitation are addressed by the ability of either participant to reject any arrangement that feels unfair. The assumed ability to say no is what underlies the practice of bargaining, with each party proposing various possibilities until a mutually agreeable trade is determined. In therapy, the client's ability to say no to the therapist can never be presumed. As noted by the Feminist Therapy Institute ethical guidelines, "a feminist therapist acknowledges the inherent power differentials between client and therapist . . . [and] does not take control or power which rightfully belongs to her client" (1987). The influence of transference, of the therapist's power as caretaker and expert, is the most critical factor in determining the appropriateness of using barter. The client is by definition in need of the therapist's help, and will thus feel pressured to agree with whatever the therapist implicitly or explicitly defines as the conditions of that help. A symbolic need to preserve a good relationship with the therapist makes some clients almost prescient in their ability to determine the therapist's wishes or preferences. In addition, the therapist may have power relative to the client due to sociocultural determinants (race, sexual orientation, etc.). If bartering is at all under consideration, the client is probably at a financial disadvantage relative to the therapist, suggesting a class difference as well. Clients generally look to therapists to make the rules of therapy, including the rules about what is considered appropriate and fair.

Another transferential consideration is that barter often opens a window for the client onto the therapist's personal life. What goods the therapist would agree to accept in exchange for therapy is information for the client, and the client may well imagine the therapist using those goods and feel either solace or anxiety about her perceived nearness to the therapist through the bartered item.

Bartering involves practical difficulties as well. Therapy, like many skilled services, is expensive. It is quite common for a client to earn a fraction of what the therapist earns, annually as well as hourly. In addition, therapy is a repeated service, requiring recompense that is both relatively high and ongoing. It often is unrealistic for a client to have anything to exchange for therapy that can even begin to cover the cost. The most logical possibility is to exchange services, since another service is most likely to match the expensive and repeated qualities of therapy. However, bartering for services carries the additional complication of resulting in a dual or overlapping relationship between therapist and client. Therapists have a heavy burden of responsibility to assure that such relationships are not exploitive, and this makes the likelihood of arranging an ethical barter for services small.

Finally, it is important for therapists to examine carefully any action that is outside of usual therapeutic practices. Haas and Malouf (1989) suggest the general ethical criterion of a "well-lit room," meaning that the therapist should feel comfortable offering her choices to the scrutiny of others. In a well-lit room populated by one's colleagues, any therapist might well feel uncertain about a decision to barter for psychotherapy, and that uncertainty is appropriate.

The simplest solution to the dilemma of barter in the context of therapy is to avoid it altogether. But this response also avoids what can be a flexible and respectful response to class differences. Parvin and Anderson (1995) note that feminist therapists may be more likely than mainstream therapists to examine the option of barter "because of their commitment to work respectfully with others of differing social values and a wide forum of lifestyle philosophies and their self-imposed responsibility to provide services for people with limited incomes" (p. 62). Perhaps the question of barter, like so many questions of ethics, is not a matter of what's right, but of what is "more right." Certainly, barter that is exploitive or is harmful to the therapy or the therapeutic relationship is unethical regardless of the economic situation. Yet, if barter can be done thoughtfully and ethically with a client who otherwise might be harmed by the financial demands of therapy, it may well be a solution that is more right than to allow that harm. Seeing too many clients at a low fee can translate into longer working hours, lower quality of work and ultimately to professional burnout (Parvin & Anderson, 1995). If occasional ethical use of barter allows a therapist to see more low-income clients while feeling fairly recompensed, barter may again be the choice that is more right.

ETHICAL GUIDELINES

What makes a bartering agreement in therapy ethical? After a general warning about the risks of barter, the American Psychological Association's (1992) ethical principles offer two criteria:

> Psychologists ordinarily refrain from accepting goods, services, or other nonmonetary remuneration from patients or clients in return for psychological services because such arrangements create inherent potential for conflicts, exploitation, and distortion of the professional relationship. A psychologist may participate in bartering *only* if (1) it is not clinically contraindicated, *and* (2) the relationship is not exploitative. (p. 1602)

I would offer the following six elements to examine when considering a bartering arrangement in therapy. The first three address the matter of clinical appropriateness, the next two are ways of looking at the possibility for exploitation, and the final point is specific to barter as a form of exchange.

1. *What is the nature of the symbolic relationship, or transference, between you and the client?* Consider the possible meanings the barter may have for the client. This is perhaps the element which is hardest to be sure of and the one most likely to make even a carefully considered barter arrangement backfire. Think about how the client sees you. If you are her or his lifeline, how would it be possible to tell you, or even know, that what you suggest feels unfair? If you are the client's emotional mother, she or he may be inclined to make an agreement that puts her–or himself–at a disadvantage as a kind of gift. Bartering arrangements are most likely to be successful when the transference is minimal and positive. A more moderate but uncomplicated transference can sometimes be managed if the barter is negotiated carefully, with plenty of attention to potential problems and the client's feeling about the matter, including checking back with the client for some time after the trade. Bartering is probably best avoided with clients who have strong, especially complicated, or particularly negative feelings about the therapist. In these relationships, the probability of the client interpreting the barter as an extension of the transferential feelings is substantial. Bartering should also generally be avoided with clients who have been exploited by their caretakers; the potential is too

powerful for the client to experience the barter through the lens of her or his history.

Clinicians have sometimes used the concepts of "ego strength" or "boundaries" to think about these factors; thus, a client who has a consistently clear sense of personal boundaries or who might be described as having good ego strength is a better candidate for barter than one who lacks those advantages. Both of these characteristics speak to the client's ability to separate the barter from the process and relationship of therapy and to her or his ability to negotiate effectively with the therapist.

Another way to examine this is to think about the kind of work that you are doing with the client. The term "therapy" can cover everything from powerful re-living of traumatic experiences to friendly coaching in life skills. Therapy that regularly elicits strong feelings, however collaborative the work, is therapy that is best left uncontaminated with the complexities of barter. It is more realistic for the therapist to consider barter with clients doing therapy that is substantially practical and behavioral.

2. *What kind of overlapping relationship will be created by the barter?* While any barter situation can be considered a dual relationship (i.e., seller-customer), it could also be argued that payment for therapy constitutes a dual relationship in this sense. Barter arrangements that involve the exchange of therapy for services are inherently more problematic in terms of dual relationships than are those involving the exchange of therapy for goods. If therapy is bartered for services, the therapist becomes in effect the client's employer, which is an additional layer of relationship in which the therapist has greater power than the client. An employer by definition is an evaluator of the employee's work (and by extension, the employee her- or himself), which therefore adds an evaluative component to the therapeutic relationship, a relationship that depends on unconditional acceptance for its effectiveness.

3. *What is the economic context?* Is it clear that the client will be unduly burdened by having to pay for therapy? Barter that is financially unnecessary is ethically dubious and probably symbolically significant, either transferentially (if the client is suggesting the barter) or countertransferentially (if the therapist is urging it). The therapist should first consider the possibility of lowering the client's fee or

seeing her or him for free, although these solutions may be inadequate, as discussed above.

The economic context includes the client's familiarity and comfort with barter as a means of economic exchange. If a client is unfamiliar with bartering, the possibilities of a mistake are greater, as is the case with any new undertaking. A client who, because of geographic or other cultural factors, is at home with the practice can be presumed to be more able to assess and negotiate a good trade. The same, of course, goes for the therapist. A therapist who has never bartered before might do well to practice on neighbors before arranging trades with clients.

4. *What will the barter arrangement cost the client relative to what it costs you?* This question addresses the basic element of fairness in the exchange. A direct comparison of fair-market value is the simplest way to resolve this, but may not be experienced as truly fair by both parties. If an hour of therapy costs $80, for example, to barter for $80 worth of vegetables could easily mean trading the yield of a client's entire garden for just one therapy session. On the other hand, trading for $80 worth of credit at a chain of furniture stores run by a client who is cash-poor might be seen by both parties as reasonable. Most often, however, it is appropriate for the therapist to barter for goods that would be the equivalent of a reduced fee, or which would be in addition to a reduced fee.

Consider also the cost to the client in time and effort of the goods that are to be traded. In the garden example above, the client has put many hours of labor into a product that will net only a few hours of therapy at best. Some clients have access to goods at a reduced price or effort through their jobs or other situations. When these goods are traded at their fair market value, the exchange between client and therapist becomes more equitable. For example, I have bartered for clothing (at its full cost) that a client received at a sizable discount when working at a clothing store, and for shampoo (again at full value) that a client obtained at cost through her work as a hairdresser.

5. *What other power differences exist between you and the client?* These could either mitigate or exaggerate any problems posed by bartering. The therapist should look at gender, race, class, age, sexual orientation, physical or intellectual dis/ability, and so forth. Greater care is indicated with a client who is at a disadvantage relative to the therapist in multiple areas.

Notice whether the therapist or the client is the one who has the idea for barter or who suggests the specifics of the arrangement. Both are relevant factors when considering power. A client may feel reluctant to reject or change any proposal suggested by the therapist, while a client who offers the terms of the barter may feel more in control of the agreement. A general guideline is that while the therapist may mention that barter is a possibility and perhaps even areas of trade, it is usually best to wait for the client to propose the specifics.

6. *How will you handle the problem of evaluation?* As described above, bartering for services puts the therapist in the position of evaluating the client's work and, by extension, her or his self personally, a situation which is clearly countertherapeutic. Service barters can sometimes be more safely arranged through a third party: the therapist receives a service from a third individual who is paid through a service from the client.

Even bartering for goods can become problematic if the therapist is not satisfied with the product received. This is a particular difficulty with relatively personal goods, such as art or something else made by the client. It is wiser to barter for relatively impersonal items that are not homemade. I have bartered for maple syrup, for example, which is of predictable quality (it is graded) and made in quantity. Poor quality in the bartered goods can be a way for the client to express feelings of dissatisfaction with the quality of the therapy or negative feelings toward the therapist. If there is any doubt about potential quality, the therapist and the client should discuss expectations ahead of time, as well as how they will handle any disagreement about whether the product exchanged meets the expectations outlined.

Ethical decisions are best made using a process that includes both rational-evaluative and feeling-intuitive aspects (Hill, Glaser, & Harden, 1995). This is particularly true when the therapist has personal biases, such as countertransference or feelings about money, which could influence the decision. Thinking through the guidelines outlined above is a first step, but the clinician should also weigh how she or he feels at a gut level about the proposed arrangement. If uncomfortable, the therapist might consider whether the discomfort is a reflection of her or his own limitations, such as class assumptions or a personal unfamiliarity with bartering. If so, consultation and further self-examination may help to resolve the difficulty. Or is the discomfort a signal that there is some potential problem that neither the therapist nor the client has yet recognized? The client and therapist should look carefully at any bartering agreement. Do both parties feel that the trade is fair? What potential problems can be anticipated? How might the therapy or the client's feelings about the therapist be affected? Careful discussion can not only head off potential difficulties, but can also open the door for further talk if the barter raises problems in the future. In addition, consultation with a colleague is a wise precaution and perhaps the best way to be sure that the proposed barter is both clinically appropriate and nonexploitive.

CONCLUSION

In the current atmosphere of managed care, "the ethics of care may be increasingly determined by the cost of care" (Parvin & Anderson, 1995, p. 57). In the face of these constraints, what feminist therapists have known all along is becoming painfully evident: the medical model of discrete symptoms calling for specific and predictable interventions is not a particularly useful or accurate way to conceptualize psychotherapy. It has led, in many cases, to a therapy that has alleviated symptoms without healing the person. One partial response to the limits of insurance is to find alternatives for the payment of therapy. Barter is one such alternative. Clinicians who are better equipped to enter ethically and thoughtfully into barter arrangements with clients have one more way to respond respectfully to class differences, to increase availability while feeling adequately reimbursed, and to circumvent the limits of the insurance industry.

Barter is never therapy-as-usual, and the therapist should enter into it with the same caution she would reserve for any other uncommon therapeutic strategy. Bartering in the context of the therapy relationship may be complicated at best, but it is worth considering nonetheless. Money for therapy may be getting short, but there is no shortage of human pain.

REFERENCES

American Psychological Association. (1992). Ethical principles of psychologists and code of conduct. *American Psychologist, 47,* 1597-1611.
Drellich, M. G. (1991). Money and countertransference. In S. Klebanow & E. L. Lowenkepf (Eds.). *Money and mind* (pp. 155-163). New York: Plenum Press.

Feminist Therapy Institute. (1987). *Feminist therapy code of ethics*. Denver: Author.

Haas, L. J. & Malouf, J. L. (1989). *Keeping up the good work: A practitioner's guide to mental health ethics*. Sarasota, FL: Professional Resource Exchange.

Hendricks, C. G. (1979). Using a barter system in psychotherapy. *Psychotherapy: Theory, Research and Practice, 16*(1), pp. 116-117.

Hill, M. (1995). Respondent to case example of ethical dilemma, monetary issues chapter. In E. J. Rave & C. C. Larsen (Eds.). *Ethical decision-making in therapy* (pp. 78-80). New York: Guilford.

Hill, M., Glaser, K., & Harden, J. (1995). A feminist model for ethical decision making. In E. J. Rave & C. C. Larsen (Eds.). *Ethical decision making in therapy* (pp. 18-37). New York: Guilford.

Parvin, R. & Anderson, G. (1995). Monetary issues. In E. J. Rave & C. C. Larsen (Eds.). *Ethical decision making in therapy* (pp. 57-87). New York: Guilford.

Shainess, N. (1991). Countertransference problems with money. In S. Klebanow & E. L. Lowenkepf (Eds). *Money and mind* (pp. 163-175). New York: Plenum Press.

The Price of Talk in Jail:
Letters Across the Walls

Harriet Sand
Angel Davis

SUMMARY. This dialogue between former client and therapist examines the relation between money and therapy in a jail setting. It is
based on a series of letters exchanged after therapy had ended and the
client was transferred to another corrections setting. We describe differences between us in terms of money and power, and discuss how these
disparities influenced each of us and shaped our communication. In
sharing our experiences, we have begun to acknowledge and bridge our
differences. *[Article copies available for a fee from The Haworth Document
Delivery Service: 1-800-342-9678. E-mail address: getinfo@haworthpress
inc.com <Website: http://www.haworthpressinc.com>]*

KEYWORDS. Counseling, prison, jail, women, Native American, juvenile, corrections, power, money, therapeutic relationship

In a dialogue drawn from letters exchanged between former client
and therapist, we examine issues surrounding money and therapy

Harriet Sand, MS, is a doctoral student in clinical psychology who works with
adolescents in the juvenile justice system. Angel Davis is a young woman, currently
incarcerated, who has spent recent years in juvenile and adult corrections facilities.
We are both using pseudonyms in order to preserve Angel's confidentiality. We
would like to thank those who made helpful comments on an earlier version of this
paper.
Please address correspondence to: Harriet Sand or Angel Davis c/o Cecelia Scott,
37 Prospect Heights, Northampton, MA 01060.

[Haworth co-indexing entry note]: "The Price of Talk in Jail: Letters Across the Walls." Sand, Harriet,
and Angel Davis. Co-published simultaneously in *Women & Therapy* (The Haworth Press, Inc.) Vol. 22,
No. 3, 1999, pp. 93-105; and: *For Love or Money: The Fee in Feminist Therapy* (eds: Marcia Hill, and Ellyn
Kaschak) The Haworth Press, Inc., 1999, pp. 93-105. Single or multiple copies of this article are available for
a fee from The Haworth Document Delivery Service [1-800-342-9678, 9:00 a.m. - 5:00 p.m. (EST). E-mail
address: getinfo@haworthpressinc.com].

93

behind bars. Our exchange addresses each woman's relationship to money and her position in the social environment in which we met for therapy. We describe our experiences and concerns regarding money for therapy. In writing this, we each claim a voice. The client's voice, particularly as a young prisoner, is too seldom heard. The therapist's voice too seldom acknowledges its power.

BACKGROUNDS

Angel: Since I was about eight years old, I've been in this system (children's services). There has always been someone in my life claiming to care about me, but all the time trying to think of ways to get more money. I didn't really have the ideal childhood, that's a given, but it wasn't really the trouble or actions to me during my childhood that shaped me at fifteen, it was being a paycheck to everyone, always. When my father died, my mother got a check for me, my survivor's benefits. Then, at eight years old, I was put into the hands of the system. So then I was a paycheck for foster homes and a shelter/group home. Then they found that I wasn't quite "normal" and took me to a "specialist" to find out what was wrong with me. Which they never did, but labeled me "troubled" anyway. Then, I went back and forth through all of these until eleven years old. At that point, they put me at my current foster home. My mother ran off for a year, and thus began my adolescent years. When we got to the foster home, my younger brother and I were the new kids. That's what everyone called us. That's the way I felt. After I ran away at twelve for two weeks, they labeled me a "problem child." So then my foster mom got more money for dealing with me. Then they made me go to counseling, and that woman got paid, too! Everyone was earning money on my very existence. That's when I started really cutting on myself, at age twelve. I was one goddamn big paycheck. I started getting high and really drinking. I didn't care. Everyone was well set up except me.

Harriet: I started doing a practicum in juvenile detention as clinical work towards my PhD program. I was interested in talking with some of the girls in detention and learning more about your experiences and the stresses you all were facing. My supervisor told me that you would be a good person to talk with because you were about to be transferred to an adult jail on your sixteenth birthday and needed support. I thought this would be part of my unpaid practicum, but I guess he talked with your lawyer, because he later told me that I would get paid to provide counseling over at the jail, and that he'd be paid to supervise me. It was upsetting to me that you were being transferred there at age sixteen, on your birthday, no less, but how much more so to you? It took a while to set up visits, and I worried about your spending twenty-three hours a day in a single cell, not knowing when you'd hear from anyone. When I first visited, I was struck by the stuffiness of the rooms and the differences in our positions: me in my street clothes, you in jail scrubs and sandals, pale and stressed. As a counselor, I had more visiting privileges than your family, an unfair result of my quasi-professional status. I felt uncomfortable getting paid more than I'd ever been paid before to do something I enjoyed. I considered how the money could have gone towards your bail, which would have made you feel better than any support I could give you in jail. As it was, the system was hurting you and just giving you Band-Aids, and I worried that I was colluding by accepting the money. I felt powerless to be helpful; what did I know about surviving jail?

IMBALANCES OF POWER

Harriet: In every therapy relationship there is an imbalance of power, but I held even more power than most therapists. When my supervisor asked me if I wanted to work with you, he consulted me first, then you. But what choice did you have? You were detained. You held only veto power. If you decided not to meet with me, then whom? There were only a few interns, and you didn't get to interview us or take your pick. I had never counseled someone who wasn't seeking counseling. I felt odd because you weren't asking for therapy; rather, you chose to take the opportunities to talk and to leave your cell, later the dorm, which my visits afforded. Our interactions were constricted by our roles of prisoner/client and free person/counselor. I could walk into the building and leave when I pleased; you could not. I decided when to visit; you didn't know exactly when I'd arrive. Together, we chose days that did not conflict with your work schedule, but I could arrive early or late, and you were just yanked from your room or work when I came. I wore a watch; you had none. If I didn't keep track of the time, you might be late for work. I took off my watch so you could see it, sometimes. You, not I, could get stuck for a while in the meeting room if I needed to leave at the wrong time.

Angel: Our relationship was based on a lot of things all at once. The issue of power was always there. When we first started talking, you were the counselor and I was the client. That's how my whole life has been. My lawyer said it would look good if I had three counselors. I was trapped, I wanted out! I didn't want to be inside the walls anymore! When I transferred over to jail, I felt more than trapped. I was dying. The whole institutional setting was killing me inside. To be able to get a visit of any kind was good.

Harriet: I, too, was influenced by the power of the locked doors that clanged shut down the hall and of the white walls of the meeting rooms. I drew pictures of them with you. They boxed you in, trapped you in stale air with no grass, sky, trees. The jail walls became visible to me for the first time in the several years I had lived in the area. They rendered you and the other prisoners invisible to the outside, unknown to most people I knew.

Because I was not yet a licensed psychologist, it was decided that I would not testify in court. For this reason, I had less power over your fate than other psychologists who conducted evaluations. I, perhaps more than you, worried about jail staff listening to our conversations; they might think I was not a "real," "professional" therapist. My relatively young age and casual dress as well as my student status contributed to my lack of confidence. I stood out from the lawyers. I felt less powerful than them. In what ways did this influence my role as a counselor? Did it help reduce the differences in power between us? Or did it lead me to try to assert my position? Did it cause me to overlook, to some extent, the very real differences in our positions?

You were in a very difficult, draining situation. You faced the difficult tasks of handling relations with inmates, guards, your lawyer, your counselors, and your family. You struggled to come to terms with recent traumatic events as well as past traumas. My school-related stresses could not compare. You had grown accustomed to guarding your feelings; you'd had so many experiences in which your trust had been violated. I had been trained as a counselor to discuss feelings, and I'd had fewer reasons in my life to guard my emotions.

For you, support was not readily available, particularly at first, when you were in your own cell. Your family and friends had fewer visiting privileges than I. A few paid counselors came to see you, including me. I, on the other hand, could seek free support when and where I pleased.

Angel: You're absolutely right when it comes down to my seeking support. I had some people writing me, but I could tell that they just wanted to have a piece of drama to rip apart, using bits and pieces for their hunger for gossip. Coming from the small town I do, I was well talked about for almost a year. Some people still remember me. Well, actually, they remember my crime. "Hey, you're that girl who. . . . " Just those few words can rip my heart open. So, no, I couldn't seek out real support because I didn't really have anyone. I had no idea how to talk to my mom. So even that didn't seem like an option, sometimes.

Harriet: You were young and had not yet graduated from high school. I was ten years older and a doctoral student. I am white; you are part Native American and part white and prefer to identify less with white culture than with your Native American roots. My whiteness made me feel more a part of the system that locked you up and silenced us both. Your Native American roots are steeped in a tradition that has needed to protest white oppression to survive. You were labeled a criminal; I was considered a safe, law-abiding citizen.

Angel: I was learning how to adapt to institutions and how to live a productive criminal life. Not really the best teachings, but what could I do? Have them lock me up in a cell instead of the dorm so that there wouldn't be any "bad" people to influence me? Just living in a county jail has a negative impact on a young girl of sixteen. The disparity between us is quite obvious. I am locked up with two felonies on my record, and they are none too pretty, I might add. And you have a quite clean record and are successful in your schooling towards your desired profession. I haven't even been able to get enrolled in college and have only a G.E.D. to prove my status.

Harriet: Financial disparity formed a wall between us, too. You grew up very poor; I grew up middle class, white. I took for granted certain material comforts. I learned to be polite, not to fight. I learned to be a good girl, go along with what others wanted, not make noise. I struggled to find a voice, not to survive. I admired your courage, your bravado that covered your fear.

Angel: I come from the poor neighborhoods. But that stopped at eleven years old. I then moved into a middle class foster home. There I stayed and really started to seek out my own identity. Who was I? Where did I want to go in this life? What's right, what's wrong? These are questions that I never could have answered living with my bio mom. My destiny would have been chosen for me. I would've become my mother: a drunk, crazy, depressed drug addict who believes that she is stuck, that there's no way out of that life. It took about a year for me to realize that life worked differently in a middle class home. This wasn't a normal average "white" home. No, I was told I was Native American and that I had to by law be put into a Native home. Before this, I'd never met a sober Native. I'd never actually heard of culture, traditions or ceremonies. Anyway, that's how I got to know who my people are. I formed my own morals and values during the four years of living with these people. But my self-esteem always lacked. I was a half-breed with blonde hair, blue eyes, and white skin. I always felt crazy and that everything I had to say was invalid or people would discount it.

Harriet: I knew you had a lot of important things to say. The first time I met you, you were very quiet, but when we started meeting, you talked a lot. I knew you were strong; I wanted you to know your strength. I wanted you to trust yourself and make your own choices, not follow others' directives as you had before being arrested. I did not want to be the expert. How could I be an expert on your life, which was so different from mine? I wanted you to realize you knew yourself better than I could, better than others could. But how could I, so silenced in my own life, help you to find your voice? I didn't know how much power I had, but I worried about having too much. To what extent did I influence you? It was hard to tell; you were so good at hiding your feelings, particularly at first. I hoped I could help you. But I did not want to become another authority figure in your life. Could we both be powerful and grow in our work together?

Angel: You have a lot to say about this part, imbalances in power. So do I. "Things are not always as they seem." You ever heard that? Well, everything had an influence on how our sessions went. Yes, the imbalance in power was obvious. Too obvious. I, however, have fought verbally and mentally against this imbalance of power. In some ways, I didn't see you as holding that much power. True, I was and am the one locked up, but I was in a world that I got used to over eight months. You were an outsider with no real idea of how life really was. I was comfortable. You had no idea how to act, what to say. You were a long way from home in there. I had to learn to call jail home. To accept my fate, whatever it might be.

OUR EXPERIENCES WITH COUNSELING

Angel: I've had counselors and therapists in and out of my life, and in jail, I had three. I wonder, is this what lured everyone to me? The money or the publicity of the case, or maybe the feeling of doing a good deed? Everyone in my life who was taking care of me was getting paid. What do they do with the money? Go out and rent some movies? Are they happy? I was worried that you needed the money because you're a student. I also knew that seeing counselors helped my case. In the end it didn't really have any effect. But I still kept hope, though. You helped me with that.

Harriet: I have been both client and therapist in my life. I've felt pretty good about my experiences as a therapist. I've usually felt that I've developed a good degree of rapport with my clients. I remember, now, one time when it was especially hard. In that instance, there were the biggest differences in status. I worked with someone who couldn't read, wasn't white. I didn't have enough experience or confidence at that point to do more than barely begin to address our racial difference and the impacts of it. My experiences as a client have been more negative: confusing, disempowering at times, validating on occasion. As a client in one group, I felt scared like a child, unsure, awkward and uncomfortable. I can think of one counselor I mostly trusted. It was still difficult, though.

Angel: I had three counselors who all claimed to care. Funny thing, they all swarmed around like flies to crap. But I did try to use these people to my advantage. I got out of my cell, got to have some time to vent. I even got some advice on how to move on from my abusive relationship with *him*. But it wasn't what I wanted. I hated being counseled. I hated always "needing help." People always joke about stuff like that. I would laugh and try to blow them off, but their words hurt what little self-esteem I had.

HOW MONEY SHAPED OUR COMMUNICATION

Angel: As you know now, I felt I couldn't let myself trust anyone, especially someone who was getting paid. When you brought a soda, it was nice, but I was so paranoid that I began to think you were trying to buy my trust.

Harriet: I never even thought of that. I thought I was just trying to be friendly, bring you something you couldn't get in there. Did it feel like pity?

The language about money and about therapy is strange. It shapes so much. You were considered to "need help" and need "stabilization." You were considered less likely to "fall apart" or "lose it" if you "received" counseling. What about "engaging in" counseling? You were not some lump to be molded. How could counseling occur in jail, where you are hardly free to be in touch with your feelings, and certainly not to express them? What does stabilization mean? I "earned money" or "was paid" to "provide services." How does the language of "client" and "service provider" move from describing an exchange of goods to describing a relationship? I don't know how to answer these questions.

I hadn't expected to get paid (I use that term because it feels most comfortable), but the income gave me money to help pay the rent. I didn't have to go looking for another job in addition to my other volunteer and academic work. I was sick much of the summer, trying to do a lot and not getting enough sleep, what with many responsibilities and a new relationship. My visits with you were one of the high points of the year. I enjoyed learning about your life, hearing you talk about challenges and how you faced them. I admired your strength in coping and standing up for yourself in difficult times and places. I enjoyed discussing problems and biases in the system and I enjoyed discussing religion and spirituality. It took you a while to feel comfortable sharing some of your feelings and experiences. I felt honored when you did choose to share your thoughts and feelings with me. I felt I was learning at least as much as you were, probably much more. I worried that if I were learning from you, I should not be paid as well; it devalued our communication. I was gaining more than money in working with you, feeling inspired, discussing important things, feeding myself as well as you, and supporting in you what I'd like to support in myself.

I considered donating some of the money; would I set some aside for you, for later? Give some to non-profit activist groups working on behalf of women in prison? How would I apportion this money? I thought about this in detail, but continued to deposit the money in my account.

Especially given that you weren't looking for therapy, I wondered how my getting paid affected our communication. What was it stifling? How was it affecting me? I felt more important for getting paid and more professional, such a boon for a student with little power in the academic and professional worlds. How much did our differences in positions limit your expression? I wondered how much more you would guard your feelings and experiences. Did you think of me as just a shrink, not interested in you as a person, just interested in the money or in the fame of your case?

Angel: For a while, I really got to like getting out of my room, having intelligent opinionated conversations. I also got to like just listening to what you believed was right or wrong. It helped me believe that I, too, could believe in something strongly, that it was okay that I was the way I was. Looking back now, I can see the effects of my talking *with* you. That everything we talked about had a lot of meaning. You helped me feel more confident and strong, instead of confused and weak. I told you my frustrations about the injustice of the system, and how my life seemed to be filled with chaos.

But when I talked to you about all these things, I couldn't do it knowing that everything I said was being heard and analyzed from a therapist's point of view. I refused to be looked at as some crazy teenager who was a good source of money. I never really talked to you about my past or how *everyone* got paid for my suffering. I never really told you that I saw money pass between two people so that they would let me sleep on their floor and eat their moldy bread. I don't think I've really told anyone of the reality of professional baby-sitters and how they hit you and put you outside to go "play" for a while so they can go back to watching their soap operas and getting fat while five of us starved until our parents came and got us. Only my mother sometimes never came. That's when I slept on the dirty floor. This was a long time ago, when my bio mom didn't spend all her money on drugs and alcohol. Like I said, it was a long, long time ago.

I could never have told you this if I knew that I was seen as just a client, not a person. I could never have trusted you if you were closed-minded, you know what I mean? We've known each other for almost two years. It feels like longer. But through that whole time we've only dealt with money twice: when you first started getting paid, and when you asked me what I thought you should do with it. For a while I didn't talk about anything important. I felt like it wouldn't be heard by un-greed-tainted ears. I didn't want to trust someone who wasn't there because their hearts led them. I guess I was tired of everything being deluded, tainted, confused. I wanted something real that money couldn't buy. Honesty.

Harriet: I feel foolish, now, for not knowing what money meant to you at the time. What it meant to you that I was paid. I didn't know that it felt to you like everyone who cared about you was getting paid, that maybe we were all in it for the money. I never had to deal with other people getting paid to care for me, except for a few counselors. As far as counselors went, only one of them really cared for me as a person, I think.

But the money thing wasn't just an issue for you as the client in our relationship. It affected me, too. I was paid to go meet and talk with you twice a week. I was paid by the session, not the hour, so I wasn't paid more the times we talked for a couple hours, but wasn't paid less when I came late or you had to go to work early. When we only met once a week, at your request, I was paid once, and the weeks you didn't want to talk at all, I wasn't paid. I just billed your lawyer by the session. You didn't even know how much I was paid: $35 a session. A low fee for a psychologist, but high for the student I was.

When you first told me you didn't want to meet as often, I didn't know why. I thought maybe you were mad at me or sick of me trying to encourage you to talk. I didn't know it was about the money, but I figured something was wrong. I partly believed you when you said you felt sick. I wondered if you'd rather talk to the other people in jail who were going through some of the same things you were.

The money issue felt especially bad to me when you told me you thought that your social security money was being used to pay me. You didn't explain right away that you believed this was happening and that you had grown tired of your money being used in this way and didn't want to meet with me as often. When you did bring up this issue, I suddenly wondered if it were true. I'd previously thought that the Public Defenders' Office was paying me with their funds and I checked to make sure that your money wasn't being used instead. It wasn't, fortunately, though you didn't find that out until a few months into our meetings. We cleared up this misunderstanding and went back to meeting twice a week, but I worried about it for a while. I think that, on the whole, earning the money put me in a bad guy role, a role I wasn't used to taking (and there you were, certainly considered a criminal). To some extent, it felt like a burden. The money wasn't yours, but even so I felt uncomfortable thinking about the question of where money goes. The Public Defenders' Office was paying me to keep you stable in a traumatizing and re-traumatizing situation. Although some support is better than none, it felt disturbing to be paid to make you feel better in a system which makes you feel bad. It was like handing out a few pieces of candy to someone being starved. Not preventing starvation, not stopping it, but both dulling and sharpening the edge of hunger.

While I was getting paid, your bail reduction hearing, which took a long time to schedule, was unsuccessful. The bail was not reduced, and no one set aside money for your bail. I thought about how the money might have gone to you, had the system been arranged differently. The Public Defender's Office was paying me to keep you stable instead of paying to get you out of jail, something which surely would have elevated your "stability" and "mental health" more than I could have.

WORKING THROUGH MISUNDERSTANDINGS ABOUT MONEY

Harriet: It wasn't until nearly a year after you left that jail and I stopped being your counselor that we discussed this money issue in much detail. It felt uncomfortable to us both, or at least, it did to me! I thought about it myself, and you thought about it, and we discussed it a little, but not very much until now. Back then, we mainly talked just enough to clarify that your money wasn't being used to pay me. Now, it's easier because I'm not being paid, but we're still in touch.

Angel: Back then, I talked to you a bit about the money and you told me how it made your life a bit easier. I then started thinking about how greedy I had gotten. People were giving and the only thing I was in any space to give was money. Money has an effect on even those who want nothing to do with it. It's part of our economic system. If you want something, you have to pay for it. I hadn't realized how important earning money was. And it wasn't so you could own a bunch of furniture and other materialistic goods that are unneeded, but so that you can survive in the world. So that you can live life without starving, freezing, or having no place to lay your head at night. I'm sorry that I ever closed my mind so much that I could not stop judging everyone who chooses to live comfortably.

Harriet: You had much more to give than money, even in your hardest moments. In working, I wanted to do something that I liked, and I wanted to fight oppression. But it's been more than just a job fighting social injustice. I have so much enjoyed getting to know you, and not because I was paid. I have learned more than I can say. We talked about staying in touch after you were sentenced and transferred, and I'm very glad we've done so.

Angel: You helped me realize that money doesn't always kill the souls of people who earn it. That only happens when you let it. Through communication, we moved past this obstacle. Through being honest and open-minded, we learned from each other. We grew up differently but felt common feelings. If we look at both sides, we will come to a conclusion that it's all right to trust each other, even if they're getting paid, or are in prison. That if you look past all the surface crap, you'll find another individual, with so much to say, so much to teach and also learn.

I think that all people of every race, age, professions, histories have imbalances in power. It's only closed-mindedness that makes it so people can't look past this. We have talked some about it, but it doesn't seem to be such a big problem now. I believe that I've been able to see past a lot of our differences so that I might look at our commonalities. I think we can/have opened our eyes to these.

Harriet: I think it's an ongoing process. I don't think we can get *past* differences in power and differences in experiences. I think we can keep struggling with them and trying to understand them, and connect in doing so. But the differences don't go away. I'm no longer getting paid, but you've told me more about yourself than I've told you, though you're getting to know me better. You are still locked up, and I am not. I wish you could edit this as much as I can, but you can't. You're still behind bars, and will be for a few more years. But you are growing inside despite the ongoing struggles you face, and you will have much to look forward to when you are finally released.

Private Practice
with a Social Conscience

Joan Fisch

SUMMARY. A clinician describes her involvement in a non-profit organization that provides low-cost psychotherapy using the volunteer services of clinical social workers in private practice. *[Article copies available for a fee from The Haworth Document Delivery Service: 1-800-342-9678. E-mail address: getinfo@haworthpressinc.com <Website: http://www.haworthpressinc.com>]*

KEYWORDS. Private practice, low-cost psychotherapy, pro bono services

As a Jewish, feminist, clinical social worker I struggle with my decision to work in private practice. How do I reconcile my desire to work autonomously and have a comfortable income with my commitment to professional ethics and religious values that emphasize the importance of addressing the needs of people who are marginalized and of working to promote social change? Have I "sold out" by making a choice which excludes my working with those who are financially disadvantaged? The ongoing tension has been eased–but

Joan Fisch, MSW, BCD, is in private practice in Menlo Park, California, and is a member of the Clinical Faculty in the Department of Psychiatry and Behavioral Sciences, Stanford University School of Medicine.

Address correspondence to: Joan Fisch, MSW, 1300 University Drive #6, Menlo Park, CA 94025.

[Haworth co-indexing entry note]: "Private Practice with a Social Conscience." Fisch, Joan. Co-published simultaneously in *Women & Therapy* (The Haworth Press, Inc.) Vol. 22, No. 3, 1999, pp. 107-109; and: *For Love or Money: The Fee in Feminist Therapy* (eds: Marcia Hill, and Ellyn Kaschak) The Haworth Press, Inc., 1999, pp. 107-109. Single or multiple copies of this article are available for a fee from The Haworth Document Delivery Service [1-800-342-9678, 9:00 a.m. - 5:00 p.m. (EST). E-mail address: getinfo@haworthpressinc.com].

by no means eliminated–by my involvement as a therapist and board member in an organization that provides low-cost long-term psychotherapy to those who would otherwise not receive the help they need. Writing this is one way to let others know about this creative way of providing community service. My hope is that other feminist therapists in private practice will be inspired to find ways to provide similar services in their communities.

Social Work Psychotherapy Providers (SWPP), modeled after Social Work Treatment Services in Los Angeles, is incorporated as a non-profit charitable organization and governed by a board of directors. The members of the board, the executive director, and the therapists are licensed clinical social workers who have been in private practice for a minimum of five years. SWPP provides an opportunity for clinicians to join together to provide a *pro bono* community service within the context of their private practices. Fees collected from clients pay the executive director's salary and other administrative costs. Policies and procedures are designed to protect the integrity of the client-therapist relationship.

A prospective client's first contact is with the executive director who determines financial and clinical eligibility and matches the client with an appropriate therapist. In order to be seen by an SWPP therapist, a person needs to be functioning at a level that will allow her/him to use once-a-week psychotherapy. Fees are based on a sliding scale and range from $10 to $45. Currently, the majority of clients pay $10 per session. The top fee is intended to dovetail with the lowest fee many clinicians are willing to charge. If the client's financial situation improves, s/he can talk with the therapist about becoming a private client.

Once the client and therapist have met and agreed to work together, the client has no further contact with the executive director. Therapy sessions take place in the therapist's office. All decisions about the therapy–when to meet, what to work on and the length of treatment–are made by the therapist and the client. The therapist is responsible for keeping clinical records, collecting the fee (made payable to SWPP), and sending it to the office. The majority of therapists see one SWPP client at a time. The executive director is available to therapists for consultation as needed.

Each year, SWPP holds a meeting to give therapists an opportunity to get to know one another, to talk about the issues that are raised in providing *pro bono* services, and to recognize collectively the work that we have done. SWPP has been well-received by clients, participating therapists, and those in the community who make referrals. The services that SWPP therapists provide, while limited in scope, do make a difference. Social change occurs gradually through the continued individual and collective efforts of all socially conscious individuals. In the words of my Jewish ancestors, "It is not up to you to complete the work. Neither are you free to desist from it" (Pirkey Avot 2:21).

My participation in SWPP has been very rewarding at many levels. I have the opportunity to use my clinical expertise to do community service. I experience a deep sense of satisfaction from my work with clients, clients that I would otherwise not have gotten to know. In the beginning I was concerned that I would think differently about my SWPP clients in a way that would be detrimental to the therapeutic process. This has not happened. Instead, I have become aware that being clear with myself about the decision to volunteer my time as a member of SWPP, rather than to accept low fees on my own, leaves less room for resentments to grow. The opportunity to work with my social work colleagues in providing this service has increased my sense of belonging to a community and decreased the isolation that I have sometimes felt as a private practitioner. While I continue to experience conflict about being in private practice, now this is balanced by the good feelings that result from my work with SWPP clients and collaboration with colleagues who share my perspectives about the importance of addressing economic and social inequality.

REFERENCE

Pirkey Avot 2:21. *The Talmud.*

Index